A

nine
summers

OUR MEDITERRANEAN ODYSSEY
RINA HUBER

First published in 2007 by Pier 9, an imprint of Murdoch Books Pty Limited
www.murdochbooks.com.au

Murdoch Books Australia
Pier 8/9, 23 Hickson Road,
Millers Point NSW 2000
Phone: +61 (0) 2 8220 2000
Fax: +61 (0) 2 8220 2558

Murdoch Books UK Limited
Erico House, 6th Floor,
93–99 Upper Richmond Road
Putney, London SW15 2TG
Phone: +44 (0) 20 8785 5995
Fax: + 44 (0) 20 8785 5985

Chief Executive: Juliet Rogers
Publishing Director: Kay Scarlett

Commissioning Editor: Hazel Flynn
Editor: Sarah Baker
Design Manager: Vivien Valk
Design concept and cartography: Reuben Crossman
Designer: Sarah Odgers
Production: Adele Troeger

National Library of Australia Cataloguing-in-Publication Data:
Huber, Rina, 1928– .
    Nine summers. ISBN 9781921208904. ISBN 1 921208 90 2.
    1. Huber, Felix – Travel – Mediterranean Region. 2. Huber, Rina,
1928– – Travel – Mediterranean Region. 3. Cancer – Patients – Travel –
Mediterranean Region. 4. Married people – Travel – Mediterranean Region.
5. Yachting – Mediterranean Region. 6. Mediterranean Region – Description
and travel. I. Title.
    910.4

Printed by 1010 Printing International Limited in 2007. Printed in China.

Author's note
Distances at sea are always given as nautical miles:
1 nautical mile = 1.852 km or 1.151 miles.
Some of the names in the book have been changed.

contents

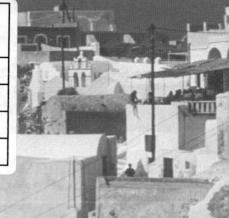

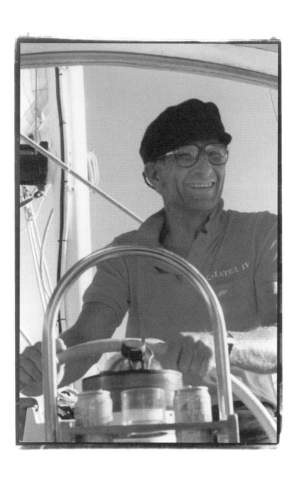

for felix
1927–1999

◎◎◎◎

Our two souls therefore, which are one,
Though I must go, endure not yet
A breach, but an expansion,
Like gold to aery thinness beat.

If they be two, they are two so
As stiff twin compasses are two,
Thy soul the fixed foot, makes no show
To move, but doth, if th'other do.

And though it in the centre sit,
Yet when the other far doth roam,
It leans, and hearkens after it,
And grows erect, as that comes home.

◎◎◎◎

From 'A Valediction: forbidding Mourning'
by John Donne, 1572–1631

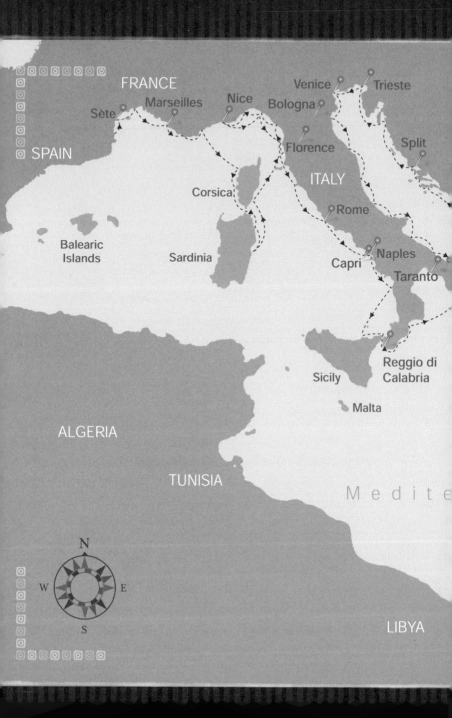

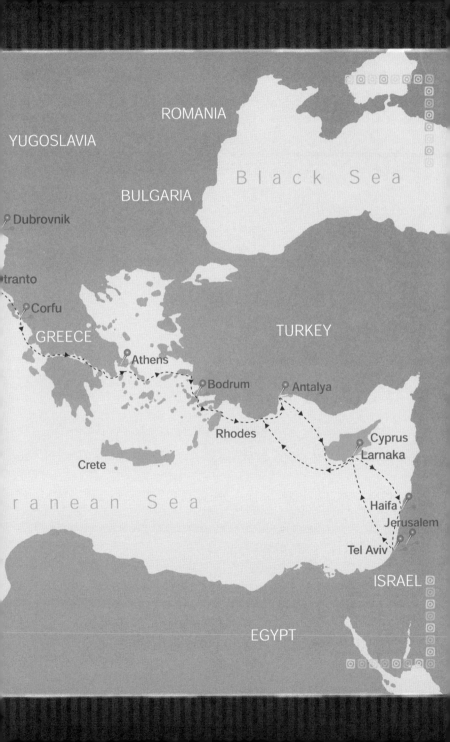

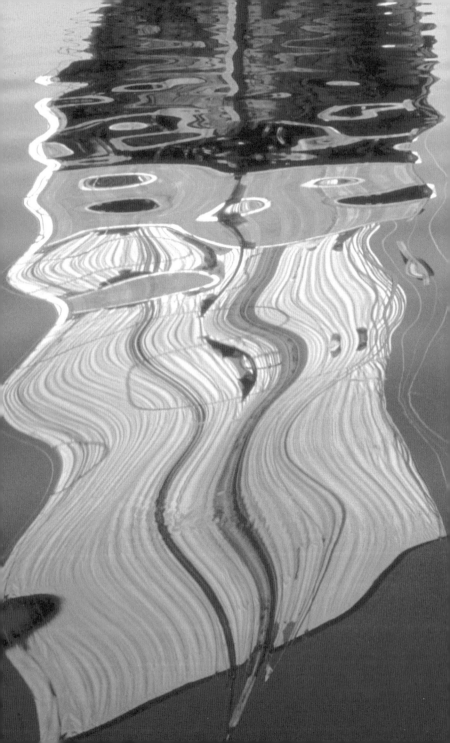

chapter one

'Three consultants can't be wrong,' I said.

'I know,' Felix said, 'but I'll be glad to have a biopsy confirm it.'

We parked the car and went to Admissions.

'Next, please.'

A woman smiled and pushed a bundle of papers across the desk. 'You're on the list for tomorrow morning, I see. Would you sign these forms please, Dr Huber. Dr Hollows's secretary has already arranged it. You're in room 317.'

We took the lift to the third floor and walked into a four-bed ward. 'I might as well get into bed, the night shift has already come on.'

A nurse walked in. 'I'd like to take your blood pressure and temperature, Dr Huber, then I'll leave you alone.'

'Sure.'

As soon as she'd walked out, a cheerful young doctor came in.

'Good day, Tom, so you'll be knocking me out?'

'Sure am, Felix! What's this I hear about you?' Then turning to me, he said, 'Hello, Mrs Huber.'

'Hi. You'll look after my old man, won't you?'

'You bet I will.'

'I'll go now, be back in the morning,' I said to Felix. 'Oh, by the way, what time shall I pick you up?'

'He's first on the list, Mrs Huber, shouldn't take long. I expect he'll be awake and raring to go after 10,' Tom said.

'Great, I'll be here.' I kissed Felix, then left him and his anaesthetist to chat.

Tuesday morning was bright sailing weather. I put on jeans and a T-shirt, and collected clothes for Felix in case he wanted to go for a sail after I picked him up.

He was still asleep when I walked into his room. I kissed him. He opened his eyes.

'How do you feel, honey?'

'Fine. What time is it?'

'10.30.'

He closed his eyes again. I sat next to his bed and waited. When he woke, he looked agitated, wanting to know the time again.

'Going on 11.30.'

From the corner of my eye I spotted Dr Hollows in a green operating gown with a mask around his neck. He was bent, walking slowly down the corridor towards us. His face looked like bad news. I felt my throat dry, my heart pound. I wanted to get up, but couldn't. He came in and sat on Felix's bed, took his time, then said, 'I'm sorry, Felix, it's not good. Retro-orbital lymphoma. I couldn't believe it. I was convinced it wouldn't be anything serious.' Fred looked devastated.

Felix stared at the bare wall opposite. Said nothing.

The clanking of a hospital trolley broke a long silence. A confused smell of coffee and hospital food drifted in from the corridor. A plump woman in a white cap and blue uniform popped her head in. 'Would you like tea or coffee, sir?'

Felix didn't answer, but turned to Fred. 'So where do we go from here?'

Fred spoke slowly. 'I guess you know the score as well as I do. I suggest radiotherapy to the area. The problem is that lymphoma in that area is so rare, I don't know a radiotherapist here with that sort of experience. You'll need to find out which place in the UK or the US has the largest series.'

Felix's lips quivered. He took his time. Yes, he knew the score. He was used to treating soft tumours.

'OK, Fred, I'll get on the phone tonight. The Marsden in London, the Memorial in New York, The Mayo, Houston, Boston…See what I can find out.'

Fred got up, and squeezed Felix's hand. 'I have to get back to theatre.'

'Thanks, Fred.'

Cancer! Felix had cancer! The word rolled and spun round in my head. It couldn't be right, this must be a mistake. To me, Felix had always been indestructible. I couldn't comprehend what had happened. I didn't want to scream or cry, I wanted to hide or disappear. I should have put my arms around him, hugged him, told him I loved him, but I was paralysed, glued to the chair. I couldn't move.

'OK, I'll get dressed now. Let's go home.' Felix put his legs down and reached for his clothes. When he'd finished, I still couldn't say anything. As we walked out of the hospital, he put his arm around me. We crossed the road in silence as we walked towards the car. He got into the driver's seat. Why couldn't I make some kind of a gesture? I was numb, my mind a blank.

Then deep inside me, I saw a skinny 7-year-old standing alone at my mother's funeral in Haifa, peering through a crowd of adult legs towards the grave. As the coffin began to sink, I turned away, looked up at the sky and told myself that my mother was up there, not in that black box. I relived the emotions of the little withdrawn girl who never cried in front of others, never spoke to anyone about her mother. Over 50 years had passed since she'd died from cancer. I barely remembered her, and hardly ever thought of her — until now, as we drove home.

The scent of wisteria enveloped us as we drove into the garage. Felix switched off the ignition, turned and looked into my eyes, 'I know this is serious, but we'll cope.' He added gently, 'You and me, we always do.'

We walked down the stairs through an arch of white jasmine, past a blaze of spring flowers into our home, a place I now barely recognised. Felix walked slowly. During the previous weeks he had seemed withdrawn. In spite of the reassurance of three consultant ophthalmologists, he'd insisted on a biopsy. He must have had a premonition.

I burst into tears. He took me in his arms and led me into the lounge. 'This is not the end, sweetie. Let's sit down and talk about it. No one can tell you how long you can live with lymphoma. So much depends on recurrences and where they occur. But you can treat recurrences with chemotherapy, radiotherapy. You can go on treating. So it's impossible to say. Some people live for a short time, but the majority go on for much, much longer. Although this is serious, it's not the end. We mustn't despair. We're lucky it's been diagnosed. I'm going to phone clinics in the UK and the States tonight, and find out which is the best place for treatment. Wherever it is, we'll go there. With luck we'll have much more time than you think and we'll make the best of it. So buck up, honey.

'But the most urgent thing on my mind at the moment is that I'd love a decent cup of coffee, instead of that goddamn awful hospital stuff.'

I put my arms round him and clung to him, 'God, how I love you! You always know how to make me feel better.'

'That's my job, didn't you know?' He winked and added, 'I'm starved.'

His nervous system needed food. I spent the rest of the day brewing coffee, making sandwiches — salami, salmon, cheeses, tomatoes, chicken. Hot drinks, cold drinks, chocolates, biscuits, bananas, strawberries, whatever I could find. Dazed, I kept going. Although it was warm when we came home, I put on an old thick sweater. I couldn't stop shivering.

Felix settled down to his desk and started to make a list of people and places to phone that night.

When our daughter Julie arrived in the evening, she could barely contain her tears. We phoned our son David in London. No matter how hard Felix tried to lighten the atmosphere, a dark cloud pressed down on us.

At midnight, Felix started to phone. First London, then New York, Houston, Boston, The Mayo Clinic, on and on…His tone was so matter of fact — cool, composed, as if he were discussing a patient's treatment, not his own. He made notes. During one break, he raised his head, his face grey and haggard, and said, 'Honey, why don't you go to bed. There's no need for both of us to stay up.' Then, with a wicked smile, he added, 'I think I've had enough to eat. There can't be much left in the house.'

I kissed him goodnight and crawled upstairs. A full moon hung over Rose Bay, silver specks ruffled the water, boats swayed. In the distance, street lights glowed, houses were dark and people asleep. What did people dream? I drew the blinds, undressed and got into bed. Bitter cold overwhelmed me. Instead of wrapping myself in another blanket, I put on my old soft dressing gown, the one I couldn't bear to throw away. I hugged myself to get warm. Thoughts of our shattered future flashed through my mind. How could I live without Felix? I couldn't.

I heard him speak, then put down the receiver and pick it up again. He had that same energy and capacity to keep going whenever he had to operate through the night then work the following day.

Warm rays streamed through the blinds and woke me. Gold patterns danced on the brown rush wallpaper. Were they telling me something? I looked at the time. 6.59 am, time for the news. No, not today, I didn't want to hear the news. From downstairs came the clatter of Felix rummaging in the kitchen. I smiled. What can't he find? I put on a tracksuit, washed my face and went downstairs.

'Hi, sweetheart. I was just making coffee and toast to bring up to you, but I can't find the marmalade.'

I hugged him. 'Have you been up all night?'

'Yes, but I'm OK. Everything's organised. We'll go to London. The radiotherapist at the Marsden has had the most experience treating retro-orbital lymphomas. He's away just now, but he'll be back next week. I spoke to David. We can have their bedroom. He and Anne will move into a flat next door. It's available, and we'll stay in their flat with the little kids. I'll phone Qantas after 9 and book. I'll have to get someone to stand in for me and look after my patients in hospital.'

'And I'll need to arrange for someone to take my classes. Fortunately, I've almost finished, only two more lectures. It's close to end of term,' I said.

'So all's under control. Try and cheer up. We're going to the best place for treatment.'

'You're right.' I put my arms around him and smelt his tired, nervous sweat, as if he'd just finished a long operating session. I didn't want to let him go.

The following days were hectic.

'Mark will look after the patients in my rooms and John is going to look after the ones in hospital,' Felix said when he came home the next day.

'And I've given the students a reading list and notes to cover the last two lectures on Mediterranean Cultures, and Peter will take my tutorials on Migrant Family Structures.'

◎◎◎◎

Five days later we left for London. It was dark as the plane took off. I looked down and saw the glittering lights of Sydney below and wondered how we'd feel when we returned. Felix gripped my hand, clinging to it as if to ensure I wouldn't escape. Was this a sign of insecurity, or was it to reassure me that everything would be all right? His role towards me, towards our children, his patients, had always been that of the consoler, the healer, the one who reassured others. All his adult life he had looked after patients; he had never been one himself. He didn't know how to be a patient. My love for him verged on pain.

'One whisky and one gin and tonic.' The attendant smiled as she put down the glasses. When dinner was served, Felix was in fine form. I couldn't face food.

'Thank God, no telephone for 24 hours.' He closed his eyes. 'Isn't it lucky that of all places, David is doing his post-grad in London?'

Our seats lent back, the lights dimmed, we spread out the blankets. Within minutes Felix was asleep. He could sleep anywhere, any time. But he didn't let go of my hand.

David, his wife Anne and our granddaughters Emma and Jackie were at the airport to meet us. It had been a year since we'd last seen them. David and Anne looked worried. Felix tried to sound reassuring. The girls looked confused.

'Goodness, how you've grown! We've been missing your hugs for over a year now!' Back at their flat, we talked most of the night before collapsing into bed.

The following morning we took the tube to South Kensington and walked to the Royal Marsden Hospital for Cancer. London squares were in full autumn regalia, and squirrels scuttled among gold and amber leaves, scrambling up and down trees under a low grey sky.

As we crossed the threshold of that old red brick hospital and wandered along corridors that branched like rabbit warrens, Felix's lips quivered and my throat felt parched. A hospital for cancer is unlike an ordinary hospital. For most who enter such a place for the first time, the occasion is a marker they use to gauge the rest of their lives. I felt my heartbeat quicken.

A large rectangular hall with high ceilings and tall windows looking down onto the Fulham Road functioned as a waiting room. As we entered, the realisation fully struck me that Felix's role here was as patient, not as doctor. I gripped his hand and held it tight as we took our seats. It was a silent place where people spoke in whispers. Near us, a young man in frayed jeans and a bright red T-shirt sat alone. His face was grey, his cheek-bones protruded, his eyes were glazed. A hairless child sat on his mother's lap as he listened to a story. A young woman stroked her mother's hand. A girl peered into a mirror and adjusted her wig. The hand of an elderly woman shook as she collected a cup of tea from one side of the room. Felix and I took our seats among the haggard, the furrowed, the bald, the gaunt, the wrinkled, the worried, the fearful, the hopeful.

We, too, now belonged in this place of fear and hope and compassion.

'Dr Huber, Dr Hunt will see you now, the second room on the left.'

Dr Hunt was in his 50s. Tall and lean, with thinning hair, a gentle face and intelligent eyes, he inspired confidence. 'Do sit down.' The consulting room was small and spartan. An old lithograph of doctors standing around a bed hung on the wall. The carpet was threadbare, the walls in need of fresh paint. A single file lay on the table.

'So, I gather you've just arrived in London. I hope you had a good trip. Tell me your story…'

While they talked, I switched off, looked out the window and tried to think about Emma and Jackie. As far back as I could remember I'd found it hard to discuss serious illness, visit gravely ill people in hospital or attend funerals. The first time I was able to stand at a graveside since my mother's funeral was when my mother-in-law died. She had been like a mother to me.

I turned back to Felix and Dr Hunt as they came to the end of their conversation.

'…So we'll need to do all the tests, then we'll plan a program. It'll probably entail coming in five times a week for about four weeks of radiotherapy, but we'll see…'

As we walked out, I didn't dare ask whether Dr Hunt had mentioned a likely prognosis.

'Let's go and eat something, then take the tube to Trafalgar Square, go to the Art Gallery.' Felix avoided mentioning the treatment. He knew how hard it was for me to cope with illness and acted as if we were on holidays. I'll go along with it. At least for today, I thought.

Seven days later, we started to make our way each weekday morning to the Marsden. For four weeks Monday to Friday, I waited outside the radiotherapy treatment room and watched frightened faces sip tea or stare vacantly into magazines. And when, now and again, eyes met, they resonated with compassion. Felix grew progressively more tired and looked increasingly gaunt, his face more lined.

It was a comfort to be with David, Anne and the girls, especially as Felix could talk about his concerns with David, who at that time was a surgical registrar at King's College Hospital.

At the end of the treatment Dr Hunt did his best to reassure us.

'As you know, Felix, it's hard to give a prognosis, but I'm optimistic. There'll be recurrences, but one can go on treating.'

◎◎◎◎

It was hard to say goodbye to David, Anne and the girls. I wiped my tears. '…It'll be great to see you back in Sydney for good next year.'

The plane took off at night. Felix ate and drank as usual, then we spread out the blankets and held hands. I shut my eyes. Felix had no problems going to sleep and keeping everything under control. But my heart was pounding, my brain buzzing. 'How does he manage to be always in control, never lose his cool? Maybe that's what surgery is about? He always knows what to do next. But how is he going to solve this one?'

The cabin was dark. Through an open blind I watched a red port light blip on and off in a black–blue sky. The aroma of coffee swept past me as an attendant handed a passenger a tray. When we neared Bangkok, a pumpkin sky bathed the horizon and a bright arc climbed from the sea, heralding a cloudless day. I saw the beauty of the world as I'd never seen it before, and wondered how many more dawns we still had together.

Suddenly, Felix sat up, wide awake, and turned towards me. 'What would you think about retiring now, buying our dream boat and sailing the Med, like we always said we would?'

Ever since we'd seen the Mediterranean together in 1953, we'd talked about how we'd 'sail the Med' when we retired. That was after an old fisherman at Portofino on the Italian Riviera lent us his stubby plank boat with an ochre sail for the afternoon, and we had our first view from the sea of the coastline, the promontory, the tiny pastel-coloured villages suspended on steep hillsides, sheltered bays, dark green pines and brightly coloured boats tied to the shore. When we returned that evening, Felix looked round the bay, then said, 'One day we'll sail the Med in our own boat!'

'What a fabulous idea,' I said. 'Promise?' And the way he said 'Promise' I knew he was serious.

Felix knew how much I loved the Mediterranean, where I'd spent the first ten years of my life — the first seven in Israel, and the following three in Italy. During the many years that followed our encounter with the old fisherman, we often referred to our 'mad dream' to sail the Med when we retired.

Now, as we held hands on our way back to Sydney, I looked at Felix in disbelief. 'Oh, that crazy notion!' I thought, and didn't know what to say. Then, almost muttering to myself, I said, 'How would we deal with medical problems?'

'First we need to decide whether this is what we really want. As for the problems, we'll deal with them one at a time.'

The old fisherman's face flashed before my eyes. His weathered hands, his crumpled hat, his loose trousers tied with string, his slow, deliberate gait as he walked away and left us to his boat — I saw it all again, and felt tears roll down my cheeks.

'Of course the idea grabs me. You know it does. But my concern is still — what if we have medical problems on the way?'

'We'd always be within a few hours' flight to London, and we'd go back there for check-ups.'

'OK. And what will we live on?' I asked.

'I don't know yet. One option is to let the house.'

'What'll we do when we come back and neither of us has a job?'

'We'll worry about it then.' Felix went on, 'We can't make five-year or three-year or two-year plans. We need to cope with each problem as it comes up.'

'OK, if you solve the problems, I'll go along.'

'You realise you'll need to do courses in navigation, radio, radar, survival at sea and all the rest,' Felix said.

'OK.'

But I continued to think about problems that to me seemed insurmountable. Felix countered them with 'It's not quite like that…' Finally, when we felt as if we'd been through all the problems and solved them, that unremitting sense of doom that had been weighing on us lifted. A ray of sun lit our faces. We looked at each other and beamed. A new life. We'd decided on a new life!

◎◎◎◎

I was alone at home when my cousin Nick and his wife Agnes walked in some days after our return. Their expressions registered a gale force wind.

'Felix told me that you're buying a bigger boat and that you're going to retire in a few months and sail the Mediterranean. Is this serious?' Nick blurted. 'Are you happy to do that, or are you just doing it for Felix?'

'Oh, no! I'm thrilled to do that,' I said.

'Don't you think you're both a bit reckless?'

'What's life about? Especially when you know it's likely to be cut short,' I started, but Nick interrupted me. 'Sure, one should make the best of it, enjoy as much as you can, but within sensible limits. What happens when you need medical treatment and you're on a boat?'

'We could do what most people would expect us to do — go on working as normal, interspersed with bouts of treatment until the end. The other choice is to do what we'd always hoped to do when we retired. Instead of waiting, we've decided to do it now. If we don't do what we want to do now, there won't be another chance.

'It's a choice between adventure and freedom or just waiting to die. Sure, there'll be times when we have medical problems, fear, depression. I know I'll be terrified when we're caught in storms. But you could say we've chosen one last adventure, to live our dream.'

There was a long silence. Agnes looked stunned, uncomprehending, but Nick was almost convinced.

A week after our return from London, we walked into a shipbroker's office. The broker was on the phone for a long time. When he'd finished, he spun his chair and said in an impatient tone, 'And what can I do for you?'

'What we're looking for is as rare as hen's teeth, I know,' Felix started, 'but we're looking for a "Savage 42".'

The shipbroker's eyes widened, and he sat up.

'That's very interesting. The bloke I was just talking to phoned from Brisbane. He's selling one, the original one Jack Savage built for himself. If you're really interested, we could fly up to Brisbane on the weekend and have a look at her.'

We stared at each other, said nothing. Then Felix turned towards him and said, 'OK. This weekend.'

For the rest of the week, we talked of nothing else. I waved as Felix backed out of the garage to drive to the airport. 'Good luck!' I called out.

'I'll phone as soon as I know anything.' To pass the time, I busied myself baking.

At lunchtime, Felix phoned. 'We've got her! She's beautiful. Needs a few minor alterations and a name change. A crew can deliver her to Sydney next week.'

It was a crystal morning the Sunday she slipped into Sydney Heads, a gleaming white hull with billowing sails, making a triumphal entry past a swarm of boats as we gazed through binoculars from the peak of South Head. Our last boat, I thought.

'What shall we call her?' Felix asked.

As we'd always chosen names from Greek mythology, I said, 'I'd like her to be *Galatea* after the sea nymph, and turn her into our dream boat.'

We followed her with our binoculars, watched the crew take down her sails and motor into the Cruising Yacht Club in Rushcutters Bay.

'I think I'm dreaming.' I clutched Felix's arm.

The crew looked tired. 'We sailed on one tack all the way from Brisbane. She's a beauty, sails like a dream. The only mishap was the television. It flew out of its locker and crashed onto the floor. It'll need repairs. Sorry about that.'

We cracked a bottle of champagne and toasted, 'To *Galatea*. May God bless her and all who sail in her.'

'Cheers!'

The crew packed up and left, and our real excitement set in. We opened hatches, raised floorboards, looked into the bilge, tested the radio and opened the refrigerator, the deep freeze, the portholes.

A 'Savage 42' had been our dream boat since we'd inspected one five years earlier. Some were sloops (with one mast), but ours was a ketch (two masts), which we thought ideal for the cruising we intended to do. The centre cockpit made me feel protected on all sides. I also liked the idea of an aft cabin, a 'bedroom', with its adjoining tiny shower, a sink and head (toilet). Apart from a comfortable central saloon, there was a forward cabin with two bunks and an additional large shower, sink and head.

'We must make a list of what we need to make this a proper home,' I said. Felix started, '…more shelves for books, for tapes, hanging space for clothes, a microwave, a spot for a computer, a printer, wine storage, locker for the photographic gear, sound system, clear wall space for pictures. New seat covers…'

'And how about sailing up to Smith's Creek next weekend and introducing *Galatea* to our favourite spot,' I said.

For almost 30 years, first with the children and later alone, we'd spent weekends and holidays on our various boats in the bays and inlets of Broken Bay, fjord-like cruising waters about 28 km north of Sydney.

So, on the following weekend, we made for Smith's Creek. We dropped an anchor near the aged ghost gum that had grown old with us. There, the scent of eucalyptus leaves, the sea breeze and tranquillity shrouded us.

That first morning on *Galatea* was bright but cold. We rolled down the plastic sides of the cockpit cover and basked in the warmth. We breakfasted on porridge with brown sugar and coffee, and watched the mist curl and rise.

'Do you remember how we used to row ashore to collect oysters with the kids, and how the family of ducks liked to come on board and demand crumbs?'

'We've had such good times.' Felix put his arm round me.

In the evening we lit the paraffin lamps, and the saloon glowed with warmth in the amber light. We played quiet music, had dinner, drank wine and listened to the night sounds of the bush — frogs, crickets, jumping fish, the breeze in the trees.

In the early morning, the water was as still and smooth as glass, mirroring the hills, the hull, the masts and the trees. It was hard to tell where image and reality merged. Two kookaburras perched on the crosstrees and laughed. We waved to them. They looked down with disdain.

That weekend was our introduction to living on board our new *Galatea*. Yes, we could live like this, just the two of us, marooned from the real world.

When we sailed back to Sydney at the end of that weekend I knew we'd never go to Smith's Creek again.

◎◎◎◎

'Perhaps we should have a long trial run before we ship *Galatea* to the Mediterranean, maybe sail to the Barrier Reef. We could do the race to Mooloolaba with crew, that'd get us up north quickly. From there we'd be on our own. It's an opportunity for you to practise navigation and use the radar and radio,' Felix said.

'But I hate big boat racing,' I said.

'Yes, I know you do, but the more time we spend on *Galatea* before we ship her overseas the better. Give it a think, honey!'

The following morning I was in a good mood.

'I've been thinking about the race to Mooloolaba,' I started. 'It sounds OK, so long as the crew isn't paranoid about winning.'

'That's good, you'll enjoy it.' Felix wasn't as enthusiastic as I'd expected.

'We'll talk about it tonight.'

When he came home that evening, Felix looked distressed.

'What's wrong? I can tell, something's wrong.'

'Don't get all upset. Let's have coffee first.'

'No. Tell me what's wrong!'

'Well, sit down.' I fell into the nearest chair.

'I had a lump in my neck removed a couple of days ago under local anaesthetic. I just got the pathology result — it's a recurrence.' I started to shake.

'Honey, don't! This is likely to happen more than once. We'll have to cope.'

'Does this mean that it's back to London?'

'No, I had a meeting with oncology and decided on chemotherapy for six months, six weekly.' He tried to reassure me: 'We won't let it change anything.'

I burst into tears. 'How can you think of racing? You'll be in the middle of chemotherapy, you'll feel sick.'

'Some chemotherapies make you more sick than others.'

'In that case we shouldn't sail to the Barrier Reef as we'd planned. The whole thing seems mad to me.'

'We can still continue north after the race. David said he'd fly up and give me the intravenous chemotherapy. That's easily organised.' Felix looked relieved now that he'd told me. 'How about we go out for dinner now?' He came over and let me cry on his shoulder.

'And don't forget about the "Survival at Sea" test next week.' This was the only course we were doing together. Felix had passed the Master Yachtsman Certificate several years earlier.

◎◎◎◎

'The test is at the Qantas pool,' our TAFE lecturer announced. 'You'll have to wear full wetsuits, boots and life jackets when you jump off the wing of a 747, and swim several laps of the pool.'

'I can't swim 30 m!' I whispered.

'I'll stay near you,' Felix assured me.

'Felix and Rina, I've arranged for you to do the test on Tuesday with a dozen young blokes who are doing the exam for their professional diploma in coastal navigation.'

As we neared the Qantas pool, I pretended to be cool, but my stomach started to churn as soon as I entered the chamber. The wing of a 747 was suspended over the water, in a badly lit cavity, enclosed by four walls and a towering roof. Flight crews trained here for emergencies at sea.

Twelve young men and a bare-footed, beer-bellied examiner wearing shorts stood at the side of the pool. We joined them.

The examiner's voice boomed. 'You'll climb up to the platform, walk onto the wing of the 747, then jump into the water one at a time. As soon as you come up, you'll swim the length of the pool four times. When you've all jumped, the lights will go off. There will be rain, lightning, wind and waves simulating a storm at sea.'

We climbed the ladder.

'Jesus, what am I doing here? I'm pushing 60, I'm the only woman, I'm crazy!'

'OK, the first person jump!' he bellowed.

Like a zombie, I moved forward. Before I had time to think, I was the first to step to the edge of the wing and jump. My gumboots hit the water, filled and dragged me down. I touched the bottom. The life jacket floated me to the surface. I looked up and saw Felix jump.

'And now swim up and down four times!' the examiner shouted at us.

I swallowed water. I gulped for air. My heart pounded. The waves rose higher and higher. I dog paddled, I thrashed about, and somehow I found myself at one end of the pool. I turned and floundered towards the other end. Lights went out. It was pitch black. Torrents of rain poured. The 'sea' became more and more agitated. Lightning flashed. I shut my eyes. My pulse raced.

'And now I'm tossing an igloo life raft into the water. Get into it. When you're all in, zip it up. I'll turn it upside down, and switch on a gale,' the microphone roared.

Felix grabbed me, dragged me to the raft, climbed into it then pulled me in. The others followed. As they were about to zip the igloo shut, I panicked.

'Can't! Claustrophobic! Got to get out!'

'Swim to the edge, get him to pull you out!' Felix yelled as he pushed me out of the raft and into the water. I fell into thick blackness and tossing waves. I gasped for air, thrashed towards the edge and caught the examiner's foot.

'Drowning!' I panted.

'Get back or I'll fail you!' he bawled, as he kicked me and pushed me back. In that split second, a flash of lightning lit the chamber. He saw me, realised that I was about to pass out, knelt and pulled me out.

I never bothered to find out whether I failed that test.

For several weeks before the race, we worked on the modifications we wanted done on *Galatea*. Dieter, the carpenter at the Cruising Yacht Club, was an artist. He fitted equipment in the saloon, built shelves, racks and additional lockers, and altered the galley. Ken Evans was a wizard with the diesel engine. By the time he'd finished, he knew it like the back of his hand, which was lucky. We would phone him more than once from the Mediterranean for advice.

Although I'd finished all my courses, I was nervous. This was my first long offshore race and I'd agreed to co-navigate for practice. Felix was being gentle with me. We would take watches together so he could supervise me. After the race we intended to continue on our own to the Barrier Reef, and somewhere along the way, David would fly up to administer Felix's chemotherapy when it was due.

It was a brilliant blue day, the harbour a blaze of colour and movement as boats jockeyed for position.

Bang! The starting gun sent a frenzy of boats moving in one direction.

'We're on our way, sure looks good.' Felix beamed. 'Evening forecast is for light variable winds.'

That evening I heated a chicken casserole and rice in the microwave, followed by a fruit pudding. It was so calm, I added a flambé brandy sauce that almost set the cabin alight. 'That was ambitious. Every race should start with the smell of brandy sauce!' Bob, a member of our crew, licked his lips.

Trouble began the following morning when the radar packed up, but Felix assured us that as long as the weather lasted, and the visibility was good, it didn't really matter. On the third day it started to rain. The wind and sea were building up, and a strong wind warning, 20 to 30 knots, came on the air. The boys furled the main and headsail to half size. When a renewed strong wind warning came on the radio some hours later, we headed out to sea. As we neared Cape Byron on the following day, a 24-hour gale warning was issued.

I was seasick, took antinausea tablets every three hours and offered them all round. Steve, another crew member, was vomiting incessantly. Tea and biscuits replaced my cuisine.

The gale still raged when we were 3 miles east of Mooloolaba, north of Brisbane. We radioed the Coast Guard for instructions.

'*Galatea, Galatea*, this is Coast Guard Mooloolaba. You'd better anchor in 10 m of water and wait for the seas to abate. It's impossible for us to lead you over the bar in these conditions. One boat's already capsized trying to cross the bar on their own.'

We anchored in 10 m, put out 50 m of chain, and sat out the gale for fourteen hours, battered by the wind and the waves. For much of the night, three of us hung over the rails.

'For Chrissake! Vomit away from the wind!' Felix shouted.

At 10 the following morning, the Coast Guard came on air: '*Galatea, Galatea*, Coast Guard Mooloolaba here. It's OK for us to come out now and guide you over the bar. Just follow us. Do you read us?'

'Roger, Roger, Coast Guard, this is *Galatea*, we read you.'

The tension was palpable. What stomach I still had was in my boots.

'Everyone put on life jackets!' Felix's tone was stentorian. We followed orders. Nick turned on the engine, and Felix took the helm.

The Coast Guard Rescue boat approached us and turned. Felix followed close behind. We crossed the bar and entered calm waters.

Exhausted, we threw our lines to people on shore.

'Gentlemen, welcome to Mooloolaba!'

'*Gentlemen*,' I muttered, 'bloody typical.'

Several boats had already tied up at Laurie's Marina. The saloon was a mess of wet clothes, spilt tea, milk, biscuits, fruit peels, sticky crockery, wet towels and rubber boots. The bunks were littered with blankets, sleeping bags and wet pillows. The place stank of vomit.

'It's been a rough trip, kid.' Felix gave me a hug.

I wanted to cry.

The crew left us the following morning. We cleaned up. Felix took the radar and torn sail to be repaired, and fixed the rest of the broken gear.

'How often do you think we'll have to sail through the night?' I asked. Ports along the Queensland coast were few and far between. Felix knew I was scared.

'I promise that whenever possible we'll shelter in a bay or behind a headland for the night,' Felix assured me. 'But we'll have to leave Mooloolaba in the afternoon and sail through the night in order to reach Sandy Straits on an incoming morning tide so we can cross the bar. We can't avoid that.'

We cast off at 4.30 pm, and settled into the routine we'd planned. We watched the sun set and had tea. As the sky darkened, lights came on along the coast. At 10 o'clock we started to split watches. Felix went down first, so that he'd be on watch when we had to change course and make for the bar.

'Well, this is it, kid! I know you're worried, but your navigation is great, and you can always wake me if you get worried.' He gave me a kiss and a big hug.

Alone in the cockpit on my first night watch, I followed a full moon rising into the winter sky, listened to the hissing of the sea and the whispering silence. A cool breeze brushed my cheeks, I tightened my scarf, pulled down my beanie and zipped up my jacket. As lights along the coastline faded, the Milky Way appeared so bright and low above me, I reached out to touch the stars. Moonbeams and stars glittered and danced on silver

30

water. In a world so unfamiliar, I lost all sense of time, of place, of reality. I felt drugged, hypnotised, as *Galatea* drifted inexorably into a surreal world, where the line between water, air and sky blurred into a circular universe.

And so we sailed on, deeper and deeper, until the lightest of pink lined the eastern horizon. The moon had set and night was giving way to a bright morning when Felix announced, 'Double Island Light is now abeam 3 miles west.'

We cleared Wolf Rock, furled our mizzen and half the headsail, and changed course to make for the bar. We sighted the Widebay Bar leads, followed in on a moderate swell, and motored to Gary's Anchorage. A large turtle swam alongside us.

In the late afternoon, the muffled sounds of children playing drifted towards us from a narrow sandy beach on the other side of the water. A dog of indeterminate parentage barked and chased gulls. A breeze stirred the fragrance of gum leaves and rippled the surface of the water. Two cormorants sat motionless on a rock. In the distance, a wisp of smoke rose from a barbecue beyond the trees. At sunset, shoals of fish flitted past, and when the moon rose after dark, we heard flying fish smack the water and watched phosphorescence glow.

From this point we started on our daily routine, preparing for the next day — plotting our courses, entering and checking these into the satnav, re-reading instructions in the pilot books, and talking to a marine communication station on morning and evening radio schedules.

The evening before our departure from Pancake Creek, we went through our usual routine and set the alarm for 4.30 am. It was mid-winter, and dark by 5.30 pm. Bent over the chart table, Felix said, 'We'll need to start early to reach Capricorn before sunset. The forecast is for a sou'westerly, 15 to 25 knots, which should reach us during the morning.

That's just perfect. If we start at 5 we should cover the 40 miles before dark.'

'So I guess we'd better get to bed soon.'

It seemed as if we'd just gone to sleep when I heard Felix whisper, 'Time to get up, kid. I turned off the alarm, to save you the shock. Here's the hot chocolate. We'll need to move, it's blowing a northerly, not very strong, but it's supposed to change to a southerly later on.'

It was still dark when we weighed anchor, motored out and set the autohelm onto our northerly course. I prepared a light breakfast. An unexpected 10-knot nor'easterly was blowing.

'We'll motor until the sou'westerly gets here. We must get to Capricorn in the early afternoon.' Meanwhile the eastern sky had turned into bright pinks and orange, but it was bitterly cold and the wind shrieked through the stays. We continued beating into the wind for three hours. I was frightened.

'I have a feeling the northerly's building up. No sign of the southerly, it should have reached us by now. Don't like the look of the clouds much, either.' That's all Felix had to say to make my heart miss a beat. Minutes later I was gripped by a blinding migraine and uncontrollable vomiting. As the wind and waves howled around us, Felix came down every few minutes to guide me to the head to vomit. I couldn't open my eyes and invariably missed the mark.

'Dear God, please let me die...'

Galatea tossed from side to side, plunging and rising from trough to trough. Felix said something about finding shelter, '...but there's nothing I can see on the charts near here...we're about 10 miles east of the northern entrance to Gladstone. According to the pilot book it's a tough channel to negotiate without local knowledge. Maybe Air-Sea-Rescue could advise us.'

I heard him turn on the radio.

'Air-Sea-Rescue Gladstone, this is *Galatea*. Golf Alfa Lima Alfa Tango Echo Alfa, Victor Juliet, Five Four Nine Four, calling for assistance. Our position is 10 miles east of North End. We're battling the northerly. Can you suggest shelter near here? Over.'

The reply was instant. '*Galatea*, *Galatea*, this is Ranger, Air-Sea-Rescue Gladstone. I read you loud and clear. Make straight for North End, and when you get close I'll guide you in on the VHF. You'll see me on the beach in a red inflatable. Do you read me?'

'Thanks, Ranger, I read you loud and clear, am changing course and heading for North End, *Galatea* out!'

Felix altered course and made for land. The change was dramatic. *Galatea's* motion steadied, and with the sails eased, spray flying and waves breaking over her starboard beam, she sliced through the water and raced towards shore. Mirroring her mood, I stopped vomiting and crawled into the cockpit. It took us almost two hours to reach North End and see the beach.

'I can see you, *Galatea*, keep on your present course!'

We could now see Ranger's red inflatable on the beach with 'Ranger Air-Sea-Rescue' writ large on its side. As we approached the shore, the wind direction changed again. It was now directly from behind. The ebbing tide, however, was moving against us.

'And now, *Galatea*, don't follow the leads, just turn to port and head directly for my inflatable!'

'Ranger, did I read you correctly? Did you say we should turn to port? According to our charts there isn't enough depth for us.' Felix looked worried.

'Don't worry about the charts, this is a channel the locals use. Just follow my instructions, you're doing fine,' Ranger replied.

With much trepidation, Felix turned away from the leads and made towards the Ranger's inflatable. The water was getting shallower, the channel narrower. We had rocks to starboard and a sand spit with waves breaking over it to port. I was on deck, glued to the depth meter.

'We'll be aground at this rate!' I shouted. 'Four metres, 3.60…3…2.50…THE MAN'S A NUT!' And at that split second we felt a thud. *Galatea* was aground. The tide was running out fast. Soon we'd be on our side.

'We're aground!' We shouted to Ranger.

'No, you're not.' he replied.

'Bloody oath we are!'

'I'll come out and tow you over the bar.'

'Quick, send out a Mayday!' Felix yelled.

I rushed down. 'Mayday, Mayday, Mayday, this is *Galatea*: Golf Alfa Lima Alfa Tango Echo Alfa, Victor Juliet, Five Four Nine Four, 13-m (42-ft) ketch, two people on board, aground at the north entrance to Gladstone in danger of going on the rocks. Requesting urgent assistance.'

'Look right behind you and you'll see us,' was the instant reply.

We turned and saw a large flat-bottomed tourist barge a short distance from us. People were hanging over the side, mesmerised by the ongoing drama.

'We've been following the instruction of this Ranger Air-Sea-Rescue and this is where it's landed us!' Felix shouted.

'You weren't taking instructions from Charlie in his red dinghy, were ya? He's not Air-Sea-Rescue, he's a lunatic. He's in and out of the loony bin!'

The crew on the barge had already put down a speedboat. In minutes they were alongside, and took our anchor as far as they could out to windward. Fortunately it gripped.

'Sorry we can't stay with you, but with this tide running out, we'll be aground ourselves.' The two men sped back to their barge. It was soon out of sight on its way in to port.

I was freezing and terrified. Charlie had gone back to his tent on the beach. Soon it would be pitch dark. What if he tries to board *Galatea*? Although the anchor held, we were tilting more and more onto our starboard side.

Suddenly, the radio speaker came alive. '*Galatea*, *Galatea*, this is Gladstone Air-Sea-Rescue. We'll send out our pilots to guide you in. But you'll have to wait till 10 this evening when the tide turns.'

'I want someone out NOW!' I shouted into the radio. 'There are just the two of us!'

'OK, *Galatea*, we'll come out now and wait with you. But it'll take us at least half an hour to motor out to you.'

It was pitch dark when the harbour pilot and his two assistants arrived in a large inflatable motor boat.

'Fancy being caught with Charlie. He nearly sank two trawlers a couple of weeks ago. He's just come out of the asylum. He's not a bad bloke, he just likes to think he's part of Air-Sea-Rescue. One day he'll really sink someone...lucky your anchor held. Wouldn't have taken much to land on them rocks in that wind...'

As the evening progressed, the wind died down and *Galatea*'s hull gradually righted itself. The men chatted, drank beer and ate nuts as we waited for the tide to turn.

'I think it's just about OK to move off,' the pilot said. 'You blokes get into the outboard, and I'll take her in.' For over an hour the pilot stood at the helm and followed the outboard as he negotiated the channel that led us into Gladstone harbour. It was a relief to tie up to a buoy and crawl into our bunk. It had been a long, long day.

Although we were exhausted, we decided to move on the next morning. The harbour pilot came alongside *Galatea* and insisted on guiding us some of the way along the channel out to sea. As we approached the mouth of the channel and were about to turn north, we heard a now familiar voice on the air: 'This is Ranger, this is Ranger, Air-Sea-Rescue, reporting for duty...'

The first couple of days we were subdued, but the weather was calm, and as we moved further north, it was also warmer. Much of the time the sea was oily smooth, the sky clear. Dolphins adopted us, dived, pirouetted to the other side, raced along or ahead and trailed in the curling wake. We turned on loud music for them. They seemed to like that. When they'd had enough, they soared away as abruptly as they had come, in search of a new game. Flying fish shot out and dived back into the sea. A flock of birds flew high, folded their wings and plummeted like stones into the water.

We spent long periods on deck, gazing at the changing colours and contours of the coast, the heaving of the sea. Much of the time the sea had a glassy smoothness as the swell rolled over an unbroken surface. At other times a breeze turned the water's surface to ripples. Once, in the near distance, we saw a long black object drift slowly. We mistook it for a container and kept a close eye on it. Sailors who say their prayers each night add '...and please God don't let us run into a container or a whale.' We watched it for a while. Suddenly, a spout of water shot into the air, followed by the arch of a mammoth black hulk, and finally a flashing forked tail.

'Wow, this is as close to bliss as one can get.' I cuddled up to Felix.

Once we heard a loud thud. 'God! We've hit something!'

We certainly had — a mass of copulating turtles — the first time we'd seen the males. They looked displeased and gave us fierce looks. The horde was so big it was hard to know which way to turn. We switched on the engine and motored out of their way as fast as we could.

It was on this — our first, long offshore sail alone — that I forged a bond with the sea. The weather was kind, the wind gentle, the silence broken only by water lapping against the hull.

Our trip to the Reef, living alone on *Galatea* and being together 24 hours a day, convinced us that this was the freedom we wanted.

It wasn't easy to find a ship prepared to transport *Galatea* to the Mediterranean. Finally, however, a Polish vessel, the *Wroclow*, agreed to take her to Sète in the South of France. All we had to do now was to let our house for two or three years to finance our adventure. But a week after we were ready to do that, we had an offer from a couple who wanted to buy it. Although the house had been our home for twenty years, the offer was irresistible. Felix phoned the children.

'…we've sold the house!'

'You what?'

'Sold the house.'

'But you never intended to sell. You were going to let it!'

'We didn't know we were selling either. But we had an offer we couldn't refuse.'

'What'll you do when you come back?'

'Worry about it then, I guess.'

Some weeks later, we bought a small flat in which we planned to stay whenever we visited Sydney.

◎◎◎◎

chapter two

We flew out of Sydney in April 1988, on the same day that the *Wroclow* sailed out of the harbour with our *Galatea* on board. Our first stop was Munich, where friends helped us buy an old car, one we could leave unattended on the road and pick up whenever we wanted to explore the hinterland of ports we happened to be in. We settled for an old Renault 9. It was an unfashionable bright blue with several dents and an antique radio. If we turned the knobs carefully, we could hear the BBC news. Music was too much to ask of it, but we could listen to our 'Teach Yourself French' tapes on its equally ancient tape player.

'This radio is good insurance. No self-respecting thief would touch it,' Felix said.

As the *Wroclow* was not due for several weeks, we enjoyed a leisurely drive to the South of France. We started in Brittany and Normandy, avoiding autoroutes as much as possible. We drove along small roads into ancient villages off the beaten track, past farmhouses, old stone buildings with weathered doorframes and bright window boxes. It was spring. Chestnuts and fruit trees were in bloom. Poplars and willows in palest greens swayed like silk in the breeze. Cows munched in green pastures and meadows were a blaze of red poppies.

Our mornings began with dunking croissants into coffee at the nearest café or marketplace, where we practised our

French with anyone prepared to listen. One morning we heard a cuckoo outside our window, but the mist was too thick to see him, and by the time the veil lifted, he was gone. Life seemed so beautiful.

◎ ◎ ◎ ◎

On our first morning on board *Galatea* I fled the chaos of the saloon, stepped into the cockpit and gazed in disbelief at the boats around us, at people on the quay, at the sunshine…just as a gull swooped over me.

'Damn!' I dived back down.

'What's the problem?'

'A bird just crapped on me! Quick, I've got to wash my hair.'

'You can't, we haven't got enough water.'

'Bloody oath, I'm going to wash my hair. And stop laughing or I'll hit you.'

'Come on, I'll wash it off.'

Welcome to Sète!

We still couldn't believe it. Along with a shipload of Tasmanian onions, *Galatea* had arrived on board the *Wroclow* some days earlier. A lorry took her to a sealed yard where she stayed for several days while French customs, who looked so important in their dark blue uniform and *casquette* caps, inspected her.

To my amazement, Felix had already learnt to argue impressively and loudly in French, his arms in full flight. He didn't have a clue about grammar, just strung nouns together and that seemed to be effective. When *Galatea* was released from the customs yard and brought to the quayside, the French wharfies wound straps around the hull and raised her with a crane. *Mon dieu!* I couldn't bear to watch as she slid and swung from side to side. No matter how hard he tried, the novice crane driver couldn't control her. The swearing in Languedoc dialect grew louder and louder. Felix shouted with the best of them, using his *haut français*.

Finally, *Galatea* took matters into her own hands and slipped into the Mediterranean right side up. What a relief to step on board, switch on the engine and motor through the canals to the marina of the Société Nautique, Sète.

We were tied up at the local yacht club, which adjoins the Mole Saint Louis in this ancient fishing harbour. Although originally we'd hoped to start our journey in Marseilles or Genoa, we were pleased to be here. The locals were friendly and, because only a few tourists came there, they treated us as a curiosity. It took only minutes to walk from the marina to the supermarket, the bank and the post office, or to drive to the laundromat, the ship chandler and hardware stores.

All around us, working boats creaked and swayed. A formation of shrieking gulls circled and squabbled over fetid bits as they escorted fishing vessels into the old port. On the decks, fishermen worked furiously, gutting fish. Whenever they motored past, the pungent smell overwhelmed us.

On the quay, a hunched man and a rotund woman in a bright headscarf stood under a yellow and red sun umbrella, arranging buckets of daffodils, jonquils, anemones, poppies and daisies. Across the road in the restaurants, waiters in black trousers and white shirts unfolded tables and chairs for the morning trade, which had already begun. Men dipped croissants into magnum breakfast cups. Whiffs of coffee drifted towards us, and loud French *chansons* filled the air.

'Hey, Puss!' I shouted. 'Stop unpacking, come and take a look. This is us in France. Our first day on *Galatea*. We're in the Med!'

Our neighbour popped her head into our cockpit. 'I am going to the baker, perhaps I can get you *une baguette*?'

'Ah *merci*, that's very kind, but we still, eh, *encore* have a baguette from yesterday.' She looked horrified. Must have been my French. 'From *hier*, yesterday? You eat *une baguette* from yesterday?' she repeated.

'*Oui...*' I hesitated.

'But *c'est impossible* to eat a baguette from *hier*.'

'Ah, *non*?'

'*Bien sûr, non.*'

'*Alors*, well then *oui*, yes, thank you.'

Our first morning, and already we'd done the unforgivable. I ducked downstairs. Felix was munching on a hunk of cheese and yesterday's baguette. I grabbed the baguette.

'What are you doing?'

'You can't eat yesterday's baguette!'

'What's wrong with it?'

'It's yesterday's. She said you can't eat yesterday's baguette today!'

'Who said?'

'Our neighbour. You should have seen her face when I told her we're eating yesterday's baguette today. Don't let her see you.'

'I won't. God forbid.'

'She's trying to be helpful. Probably thinks we're lost.'

'Do you think we should tie a kangaroo to the mast?'

'Don't need to. They know already. For God's sake, stop eating. She's bringing us a fresh baguette!'

Our masts and boom lay strapped on deck. The saloon was crowded with boxes and unpacked equipment. Felix stopped chewing, looked around and scratched his head.

'Where do we begin?' I asked.

We felt almost at home when a parking ticket appeared on the Renault's windscreen. 'Damn, some things you can't escape!' I said as I freed it from the windscreen wiper. The French instructions on the back read: 'Get stamps from the *bureau de tabac*, stick them on the parking ticket and send the completed note to the Office of the Traffic Police.'

'*C'est la vie*. What better way to make us feel accepted.' Felix was philosophical. 'You go and fix this,' he suggested. 'Meanwhile, I'll get an adaptor for the TV, and let's meet here in an hour.'

Bureaux de tabac are small shops that sell cigarettes, tobacco, newspapers and stamps. I set off to the market square, where I'd noticed one some days earlier. Practising my French on the way, I greeted the mother-earth figure sweeping the footpath in front of her shop. With her floral scarf and long skirt she reminded me of Russian matrioshka dolls that fit inside one another.

'*Bonjour, madame*,' I said. '*Je voudrais des timbres pour cela.*'

She looked astonished, stopped sweeping and studied me, grim faced, as I stammered and pointed to the parking ticket clutched in my hand.

'*Mais, non, non!*' she responded.

'*Pourquoi non?* Why not?' I asked.

She beckoned a formally dressed elderly gentleman who was perusing the day's papers. 'Ah, *bonjour, monsieur*,' she addressed him. Then she ventured into the local patois. When she had finished, he turned to me. '*Madame*, this you must not pay!'

'Why not?' I asked, puzzled.

'Because nobody pay this, it is local French custom.'

'Well, then, who does pay?'

'I think only English and German people. The Italians and Spanish are like us. What you must do is what everybody in France does. That is, you must tell your *facteur*, I think this is postman in English. That when a letter comes from the police, he must write on the letter "*adresse inconnue*", address not known.'

'But I have no address, no postman, I live on a boat.'

'Ah, in that case you just tear up, like so,' he said indicating how one tears up a letter, 'and put it in this rubbish bin.'

'Where I come from, I'd be in real trouble if I didn't pay.'

'Ah, the English, funny people.'

'I am not English, I'm Australian.'

'*Madame*, you must remember this is France, not Australia.'

I looked incredulous. He dismissed me with disdain, shrugged his shoulders, handed me the ticket and turned back to the newspapers.

'*Merci beaucoup, madame et monsieur, bonjour.*' Admonished and confused, I rushed out of the square.

Then I had an idea. The obvious person to check with was the manager of the hotel where we'd stayed for several days before *Galatea*'s arrival. He spoke good English but was unfriendly. (I realised later that, by French standards, we were far too casually dressed for an establishment such as his.) Attired in a sombre suit, he was a grim, unsmiling man with a handlebar moustache and a slip of dark hair glued to one side of his bald pate. As usual, he was standing at his desk in the foyer, overseeing his domain. I approached him, parking ticket in hand, and explained my dilemma.

'*Madame*,' he said gravely, without stirring a muscle in his face, 'you have two options. One: you can pay.' He paused to note my reaction. 'And two: you can do what I do,' and with a flurry of hands and arms, he gave a graphic demonstration: 'You can just tear it up.'

'Thank you, *monsieur*,' I said and ran down the steps to Felix, who was waiting for me in the car. I stopped in front of the bonnet, and emulating the flurry of arms and hands I'd just witnessed, tore up the parking notice.

'Are you crazy?' Felix looked dumbfounded.

'No, I'm just learning to be French!' I announced as I hopped into the car.

'And how did you get on about adapting our TV?' I asked.

'No good. The French and the Russians use the Secom system. Everyone else uses PAL, and when I asked him why, he just said, "Ah, *monsieur*, you must understand, we had President de Gaulle."'

Felix's daily routine started with a visit to Monsieur Bricolage, the ubiquitous French hardware giant. He was there on the dot of 8.30 every morning in search of gas, water, plumbing, electric and other assorted fittings. Each day his French became more daring. Unencumbered by French grammar, and with a remarkable memory for vocabulary, Felix's formula was simple — shed inhibitions and string words together.

People's patience amazed us. At the hardware store they greeted Felix, now their most valued and interesting customer, with exuberance, and looked upon each of our problems as a personal challenge. Every day they found treasures for us. 'Ah, *Monsieur Felix, nous avons trouvé...*' — varieties of plugs, switches, adaptors, pipes, hoses, elbows — all the items he needed to adapt, adjust, connect and replace.

As first assistant, my job entailed fetching instruments, holding, turning, pushing, pulling and shining torches as Felix crawled into the interstices of the engine, bilge and lockers to thread pipes and wires from one end of the boat to the other.

'Pliers! Shifting spanner! Phillips screwdriver! Not this size, next size down! Bigger torch…try to hold it steady!'

'I don't know how you can see what you're doing.'

'This is no different from abdominal surgery. You gotta *feel* kid, you just gotta *feel*.'

'What are we going to do about stepping the masts?'

'We'll need a really big crane. I'll have to ask Michel, the foreman. It may be possible to do it right here.'

But when Felix spoke to Michel, he said we could use the yard crane to put in the small mast, but not the main mast. For that, Michel said, he'd ask Louis, who had a big crane. A week later Michel reported triumphantly that Louis could bring the mobile crane to the naval shipyard and that the commander-in-charge had given permission for *Galatea* to use their dock for two hours.

By this time we had learnt that the French soul, unlike the sanguine Australian philosophy of 'She'll be right, mate', is one steeped in deep pessimistic foreboding. So to begin with, most things are '*pas possible*'. With patience, this is eventually replaced with '*peut-être,* perhaps'. When this happened we knew that progress had been made, and we were well on the way.

And so Michel, Felix and I motored out of the marina to the nearby naval dockyard, where Louis was waiting with his big crane. He manoeuvred it down a ramp to *Galatea*, where Michel and Felix had secured the straps under the mast, which lay horizontally on deck, and started to raise it slowly. Then the nervous shouting started.

'Ooh! *Non, non, un peu à droite,* a little to the right, *plus haut, haut*, higher!'

'Hold it, hold it!'

Finally, in a joint effort, Felix and Michel led the foot of the mast through the deck and lowered it gently into place onto the keel. At last it was done. Then, we raised glasses filled with Australian wine, and toasted *Galatea* yet again. 'May God protect her and all who sail on her. Amen!' Although I didn't smash the bottle onto her bow, in my large straw hat I nevertheless felt like the Queen.

We motored back to the club in great cheer. The following day the short mizzen mast was lifted into place with the small crane at the club marina.

'This calls for celebrations.'

There were many things we had to learn about living in our new environment — for instance, that shopping had to be done before midday or after 2.30, for during those two and a half hours the world stopped for siesta. At first we found it difficult to adjust. Whenever I found myself in a supermarket at 11.45, mere whispers turned into a chorus of '*bon appétit, bon appétit*', and before the church bells finished tolling midday, *tout été fermé*, everything was closed, and there I stood with only half my shopping done, looking on as the baguette-bearing masses fled home for lunch and siesta. The chances of being served decreased as the hands of the clock approached the hour. By 11.50 I was the only customer eager for attention. If I looked sufficiently lost, someone took pity on me and served me as quickly as possible, lest they be caught in the middle of a transaction when the clock struck *midi*.

Back at the yacht club, we carried on with our work without taking a break, while the winers and diners at the marina restaurant above us looked down with disdain. Presumably our Australian ensign fluttering at *Galatea*'s stern explained it all.

'How does anything ever get done around here? Can you imagine if everyone in Australia trotted off to eat and drink for two or three hours in the middle of a working day?'

Each day, however, we were less enthusiastic about working through the middle of the day, while everyone else enjoyed their siesta. After a week or so, we started to wonder.

'Maybe it really *is* true that in this climate one actually *needs* to have a midday rest. Perhaps they're not so stupid after all.'

And before we were consciously aware of what we were doing, we found ourselves rushing off to the baker for fresh baguettes three times a day, and followed lunch with a siesta. Sometimes we had lunch at the marina restaurant, looked down at *Galatea* and decided it really was crazy to work through the lunch hour.

The first time we wandered into the square where farmers brought their produce to market, we were bewildered by the sounds, the smells, the colours. Stalls laden with an endless variety of fruits, vegetables, cheeses, breads, sausages and pastries stood under bright umbrellas. We stood and stared, then took deep breaths and rushed from stall to stall. So many varieties of produce we'd never seen before. After we'd slowed down sufficiently to get into conversation, sellers realised we were ingenues, took us under their wing and proceeded to enlighten us. They gave us recipes and graphic instructions on how to prepare, cook and eat these culinary gems.

One rotund, jolly fellow, in crumpled brown trousers, braces and an old felt hat, beckoned us over to his *pâtés* and *saucissons.*

'*Ces saucisses à la languedocienne sont très très fraîches, exquisite,*' he declared, extolling the freshness of his Languedoc sausages.

'*Comment cuire*? How do you cook them?'

'Ah, *madame*,' he said, and in an evocation of a loud kiss, brought his thumb and fingers to his lips. '*C'est un rêve*, a dream. You must sauté the *saucisses* in pork or goose fat, then cook with garlic and herbs in a covered dish, *et finalement servir* with a tomato and caper sauce and lots of parsley.' It took a long time to convey all this with the dictionary and the help of people at adjoining stalls. We bought three *pâtés* and promised to return for sausages the following week as soon as our galley was usable.

At the mushroom stall, a cheerful, smooth-faced young woman, whose coarse hands resembled a 60-year-old's, explained that this was not the best time of the year for mushrooms. Nevertheless, she suggested we buy the wild variety and cook them in a fry pan with a lot of butter, some garlic and large-leafed parsley from the adjoining stall. She then demonstrated how this delicious dish should be mopped up with fresh baguette. At a cheese stall, we wondered how we had managed to live for so long and know so little of these gastronomic wonders.

We sneaked back on board, hoping our neighbour wouldn't see us.

'Imagine what she'd think if she saw us coming with this load? The next thing I must get is a straw shopping bag to make me feel more…you know, *française*. I can't walk around with a plastic supermarket bag from Sydney.'

As the chaos on board cleared, and my embarrassment whenever I saw our neighbours eased, we started to chat with them. Francis and Giselle spoke slowly enough for us to understand, and we struggled with our school French. The boat was their permanent home and they moved around to wherever Francis, a mechanic, found work. He was a quiet young man with intelligent dark eyes.

They gave us insights into French life as well as their former life in Algeria. We enjoyed their company and they enjoyed our Australian wine. They visited us often, but were never casually dressed.

'...you know, we are pieds-noirs, Algerian of French parents. Colonials. Our families went there with the first *colons*. We came here to France when we got married three years ago. We miss our family, but there's no future for us in Algeria. My brothers want to stay there, so does Giselle's married sister, but we didn't.'

'Have you always lived on your boat?'

'We bought a boat because we couldn't afford a house, and also this way we can move around to wherever I can find a job. The only trouble is that Giselle can't get work. Jobs are hard to get. She was a secretary in Oran but she can't get that sort of job here. The only other thing she could do is work in a shop, but they prefer locals. And also, because I have to move around and we live on a boat, people don't want to employ her.' He turned to Giselle and smiled, 'It means she has time to keep the boat very clean, and she's a very good cook. Especially Algerian food, *n'est-ce pas, cherie*?'

After drinks with us, Giselle and Francis always joined the promenade along the canal before returning to the boat for their evening meal.

La promenade brought Setoise and their *chiens*, primarily poodles, known as *caniches*, onto the quay for a stroll or an aperitif. As they promenaded, they checked out menus displayed in front of the restaurants that lined the canal. People stopped and chatted. '*Et comment va le petit bébé?* How is the little baby?' one woman asked another. A sad-eyed white poodle peeped from his owner's jacket to demonstrate just how ill he was.

'Have you noticed how some people sport a big white poodle, others a tiny black one?' I commented. 'I think poodles are markers of the local class structure. Those who have enough space and wealth to sport a large white poodle are higher up the class structure than those with a tiny black one.' Felix wasn't convinced.

Around 8 o'clock, people retired home or into restaurants, and the serious part of the evening commenced. The first time we walked into a restaurant in Sète, there wasn't a tourist in sight, and everyone was eating seafood, for which the area is famous.

'Can I help you?' The proprietor took us under his wing. 'You are from the Australian boat, *oui*?' News travelled fast here. We sipped *vin de la maison*, nibbled wrinkled black olives and dipped bread into olive oil. We started with fish soup into which one stirred *rouille* (mayonnaise, garlic and saffron, with the emphasis on garlic) and small pieces of bread. Louis, the proprietor, noted our appreciation. He then ministered over sea bass, the freshest grilled fish we'd ever tasted, new potatoes and a tomato, basil and eggplant dish. And for dessert, we had Felix's favourite — wild strawberries with a vanilla *crème*. We had a little too much *vin de la maison,* and slept well that night.

After almost four weeks' work, most jobs were done, and when we were downstairs in the saloon, it was almost as if we were on the marina in Sydney, or anchored in Broken Bay.

The solution to the gas bottles was in sight, the hose problem was solved, and adapting the inverter had reached the '*peut-être*' stage. Only the electrics were still in the 'too hard' basket. The relaxed atmosphere of the little town suited us — the routine of fresh baguettes for breakfast, lunch and dinner, the midi '*bon appétit, bon appétit*', the brilliant idea of a three-hour siesta. We continued to buy in bulk at the market, where a number of people now took personal interest in how our new cuisine was progressing.

'Isn't life just *great*!' I squeezed Felix's arm as he lugged our purchases along the marina.

Although our tempo had slowed down to match that of the people around us, much to our amazement we realised that we had just about completed *Galatea*'s commissioning, and were almost ready to haul the sails.

'We'll need to go to Cap d'Agde for the antifouling. It's only a short sail from here. There's a new marina with all the modern facilities there. And the girl at the office said there's a Language Institute there as well. They offer a two-week crash course in French. So shall we go and arrange both?'

'Sure, but that girl said our French has improved so much. Do you think they'll employ us as teachers?'

'Ho, ho,' Felix smirked.

Spit and polish had cleaned up *Galatea* inside and out. Our geranium, chive, basil and mint pots were tied in place, the barbecue was ready for use. Olivades cushions we had brought from Sydney added colour to the beige bunks and created a Provençal atmosphere in the saloon. In the aft cabin, where we slept, the double bunk was covered with a navy patterned bedspread with matching pillows and cushions.

Bookshelves lining the port side of the saloon were filled with reference books, sailing and technical manuals, water pilots, travel books, history books, novels and, above all, books such as Fernand Braudel's *The Mediterranean and the Mediterranean World in the Age of Philip II,* the book that had inspired our idea of sailing from port to port; Julius Norwich's books *Venice, Byzantium* and *The Normans in Sicily;* Jan Morris's books on Venice, as well as books we had wanted to read for years, such as Proust's *A la recherche du temps perdu.* There were more bookshelves in the aft and forward cabins.

Both sides of the saloon were lined with tapes of all the CDs and records we had enjoyed at home. The teak panels, the cushions, the gold carpet and oil lamps, all contributed to the warm glow of our cocoon. And with it, we hoped, to a sense of stability wherever we found ourselves. There was nothing frugal about the lifestyle on which we were about to embark.

◎◎◎◎

Then the day we had dreamed of for 35 years dawned. After four weeks, at midday on a blue, blue day, we set sail from the Société Nautique, Mole Saint Louis, Sète. We farewelled the people at the club, raised the gangplank and backed out of the berth, motoring to the exit of the harbour on our way to Cap d'Agde.

Felix hoisted all three sails — the mizzen, main and headsail — and as we turned off the engine, an enormous sense of exhilaration, tinged with disbelief, overwhelmed us. Felix put his arms around me. Two seagulls saluted, followed us a short way, then turned back to port. The sea was calm and a 10-knot breeze swept us along. *Galatea*'s bow cut through the water and, like her namesake, she came to life. Mist veiled the shore, but the sky was a cloudless china blue. A small sloop crossed our path and waved. Our sails billowed in the breeze and the chorus of 'Ode to Joy' reverberated around us as we toasted the sea, the sun, the wind and our new life with Dom Perignon.

We sailed along the flat coastline, the outer shores of the Etang de Thau until, through the haze, Mont d'Agde appeared behind the new complex that was Cap d'Agde. At the entrance to the new port, a mariner from the *capitainerie*, the harbour office, guided us to a berth.

While Sète had the aura of a romantic old Mediterranean fishing town, Cap d'Agde was new and unromantic. It was one of several marina complexes known as *ports de plaisance,* built in the 1960s and 1970s along the coastline between Marseilles and the Spanish border.

Their marinas were large, cheaper than elsewhere in the northern Mediterranean and packed with yachts that rarely left their berths. Their owners lived as far away as Paris, Milan, Amsterdam or Zurich, and visited when they could, which for many was not often. These ports had all the paraphernalia of new tourist developments which, apart from the few weeks of high season, were a landscape of near-empty tables under multicoloured sun umbrellas; sad waiters waiting for a tourist to order a drink, a pizza, a toasted sandwich; ice-cream parlours, takeaways and discos. From early morning, the scent of food filled the air. Gaudy bikinis and beachwear hung on racks outside shops lining the esplanade. With hands behind their backs, owners stood in doorways, perusing the scene, waiting for customers.

Music boomed to dispel the sadness of an almost deserted resort, which only filled with frenetic people in search of sun and fun during the summer holiday period.

'Just as well we're only here for two weeks,' Felix said. 'Let's get the bus to Sète tomorrow and pick up the car. We can visit places near here, like Old Agde and Béziers. We could also drive along the Canal de Midi.'

So, we picked up our car and parked it near *Galatea*. Two boats arrived at the same time and tied up next to us. On board one were two excitable white poodles, on the other a bad-tempered dachshund and a gentle Labrador. Felix jumped ashore to catch their lines, while I fended them off *Galatea*. The two couples were French, in their late 20s and 30s, fashionably attired in designer resort wear. The women were coiffed and manicured, the men's hair was carefully trimmed. They were polite and thanked us, then went ashore to decant the dogs, who were just as well groomed.

For the French, dressing with style is important, but they also express their personalities in the adornments they shower on their dogs. Collars come in varieties of designs, frequently decorated with studs or diamantes. For additional panache, however, bright neck scarves (often matching the mistress's) are deemed suitable resort wear.

In the middle of their first night on board, one of the dogs started to bark. Within minutes there was a chorus of howling. Soon after, we heard the couples having serious words with the animals on deck.

But it was not until we heard dogs and humans chasing each other on *our* deck that we emerged into the bedlam. I saw both couples running around stark naked, chasing dogs over and under rails.

'Oh, *pardon, pardon*,' I said, unable to stop myself gaping. Felix laughed.

Chasing dogs stark naked in the moonlight caused the dog owners no embarrassment. Their only concern was the barking. 'Ah, *mon dieu, l'abaiement*, the barking, *c'est terrible. Vraiment desolé*. Truly sorry…'

'Ah, *c'est de rien*, it's nothing,' we assured them.

'Do you think they saw anything funny in all this?' I asked Felix when we went back to bed.

'Not really. It's the sort of thing the English would think funny — *Fawlty Towers* stuff.'

The following morning they asked us to join them for coffee. The night's events hardly rated a mention.

On the day *Galatea* went on the slips to have her bottom anti-fouled and painted, we started our French classes. For the following two weeks, we spent each morning at the Institute de Langue in a class with two English women who had come to Cap d'Agde to holiday and improve their French.

Each morning we covered a new topic, concentrating on areas of greatest importance to tourists: restaurants, hotels, shops and asking directions. The two weeks passed quickly, and by the last day we felt we had learnt a lot. There was only one topic we still had to cover — a medical emergency. What do you do when you have an accident? How do you address doctors and nurses?

Felix and I were too excited about our imminent departure to take much notice, and the two English women seemed just as uninterested, so the teacher agreed to finish early. The five of us set off for a farewell drink and a final chat in French. We laughed a lot, and our teacher Madame Renard told us how well we'd done.

'Now that our French is entirely to our satisfaction, and all the work on *Galatea* is finished, the only thing we have to do is have the car serviced in Sète, and we're ready to take off.' Felix announced.

'So this is it,' I said in disbelief.

'Can we leave the car with you for a service, Madame Thomas?'

'Ah, *bien sûr*, of course.' Madame Thomas burst into a broad smile. When she wasn't sitting in her tiny office writing notes about repairs needed for cars in her care, Madame Thomas walked about with a spray bottle and a rag, cleaning windscreens. She loved her garage with proprietorial affection. She was a short and plump, cheerful woman, who knew everything about everyone. She was, we sensed, an institution in Sète.

'We'll pick up the car in a few days, when we're somewhere along the French Riviera,' we continued. 'Tomorrow we leave for Port Camargue, but we'll phone you before we come.'

'*C'est bon, c'est bon. Alors, bon voyage et bonne chance.*' She waved as we left to take a bus back to Cap d'Agde.

That evening we spent a long time looking at charts, plotting our course, entering it on the satnav and familiarising ourselves with the entry, depths and port plan of Port Camargue, our destination.

'Should we bother with the depths of any other entrances on the way?'

'No point. We're not stopping anywhere. We're going straight to Port Camargue.' Felix got up and looked around. 'Well, we've just about covered everything.'

'I guess we should go to bed now,' I said.

I tossed and turned much of the night and kept Felix awake. At 2 we gave up trying to sleep and had tea and toast, looked at the sky and listened to the latest forecast. By 4, I was exhausted and went back to bed. Felix woke me at 8. We dressed quickly, had a light breakfast, admired the clear sky, took deep breaths and looked at each other.

'I wonder where we'll be in a week or a month or a year?' I said.

'Yes, I wonder,' Felix answered.

We backed out of our berth on a bright Saturday in July and waved to people along the quay and the marina. As we motored past the entrance lights to Cap d'Agde and out to sea, a seagull perched on a yellow buoy beat its wings and folded them again.

With *Galatea* turned into the wind, Felix hauled up all three sails, then stepped back into the cockpit. I set the compass to 63 degrees, switched off the engine and put her on autohelm.

We were on a broad reach in a fresh breeze, making a steady 4 knots. The passage to Port Camargue promised to be, as the French say, *une promenade*. The sky was a misty sapphire speckled with gauzy clouds. The only sound was the hiss of water and the billowing of sails.

Flocks of sea birds drifted in circles over the beaches and out to sea. To port, a string of beaches unfurled as we sailed past. Sun umbrellas in bright reds, blues and yellows dotted the sand. Bathers on shore and in the water tossed balls and balloons into the air. Multicoloured sailboards pirouetted on waves and festive music drifted out to sea. It was a blissful summer's day.

We were too moved by the occasion to speak. After some time, I shook myself. 'Lunch?' I asked Felix.

'How about a bottle of Australian red I brought specially for today?'

'Like what?'

'Like a Grange Hermitage.'

'You're kidding!'

'How could I kid on an occasion such as this?'

'I'll bring up anything you care to mention. At the *charcuterie* they thought I was buying up the shop.'

Felix stepped down the companionway into the saloon, lifted the floorboards, hauled the bottle from our cellar and turned on what was to become our theme tune, 'Ode to Joy', opened the bottle, spread his arms and started to conduct as we sang along.

Freude, Schöner Götterfunken
Tochter aus Elysium...
Joy, beautiful spark of the Gods
Daughter of Elysium...

I cut the baguette, sliced salami, placed unwrapped cheeses and pâtés onto a platter, and prepared a salad of tomatoes, buffalo cheese, basil and oil. And for dessert, a basket of cherries, a strong-smelling cheese called Pont L'Evêque, fruit tartlets and nougat chocolates.

'Smells fantastic, even the Pont L'Evêque.' Felix stopped conducting to give me a hug. Plumes of light spray swept our faces, the sea rippled and the wake gurgled.

It was a long, unhurried lunch. We looked at each other, held hands, drank the Grange and gazed at the scene around us. When we'd emptied the bottle, eaten the tartlets and had coffee and chocolates, Felix went downstairs.

'…be back in a minute.'

Meanwhile, I cleared the plates and folded the table. The wind had steadily strengthened. I alternated between elation and fear. Can this be true? Is this really the start of our grand adventure? If only the kids could see us! I couldn't sit still. In need of something to do, I took sights and checked our course, gazed at the sea, the sky and the coastline with such intensity, it was as if I were trying to imprint every detail of this day on my mind. *Galatea* was flying, our wake unravelling like a rope.

'Hey, Puss, look at this! A steady 7 to 8 knots! What a ride!'

He didn't hear me. Where was he? Still downstairs. The wind continued to strengthen. It was now blowing 15 to 20 and we were beginning to yaw. I pulled in the headsail and the main to steady her.

'Hey, Puss, come out! See what you're missing! This is our first day!'

I stood at the helm and heard several unusual thumps. They seemed to come from the aft cabin, behind me. At first I took no notice, but they grew more persistent, as if something was loose, banging on the cabin hatch that opened onto the cockpit.

'Puss, something's loose. Something's banging in the aft cabin. Have a look!' I shouted. Surely he must have heard. I waited, then I heard it again. A persistent 'thump, thump...'

I slid back the horizontal hatch and saw Felix slumped against the short ladder and the vertical hatch. His face was grey, vomit dripping from his mouth and chin onto his T-shirt.

'Oh my God! Puss, it's you!' I pulled out the hatch board, gripped him under the arms to lift him into the cockpit. He was too heavy and started to slide back into the cabin. I bent to grip him around the chest, hauled him over the hatch rail and dragged him onto the cockpit seat. He heaved, tried to throw up, wanted to say something. His speech was a garbled whisper I didn't understand. Then I did.

'Having stroke, radio...Mayday...help...losing speech...take down sails...'

I was terrified he'd choke on vomit. I turned him onto his side and clicked his safety harness into a cockpit bolt. His eyes were closed. I panicked. Was he unconscious?

'Dear God! What shall I do?' I cried out. Then I started to give myself orders.

Mayday. Must send a Mayday! I rushed down the gangway, turned on the radio.

'Mayday, Mayday, Mayday...This is *Galatea*. Golf Alfa Lima Alfa Tango Echo Alfa...Victor Juliet, Five Four Nine Four, Position 43.28, 4.02, south of Palavas. Need immediate assistance. My husband is having a stroke!'

An instant reply: '*Galatea...Galatea, ne comprends...ne comprends*. Don't understand.'

Oh, God! I don't know the word for stroke, what should I say? Try heart attack.

'*Mon mari…un attaque cardiaque…un attaque cardiaque très, très grave!*'

This can't be real. I can't stay at the radio. Have to take down the sails. I looked into the cockpit. Felix was still on his side, vomiting onto the cockpit floor. The wind continued to intensify. I switched off the autohelm, turned *Galatea* into the wind to take down the sails. I grabbed the winch handle and rolled up the headsail.

I heard the radio again. '*Nous ne trouvons pas votre bateau. Combien de metres? De quelle couleur?* We can't find your boat. How many metres? What colour?' I tore past Felix. He looked terrible, but I couldn't stop to help him. I rushed back to the radio. Why can't they find us?

'*Treize metres, blanc, deux mâts, pavilion Australien, mon mari très très malad!* Thirteen metres, white, two masts, Australian flag, my husband is very very ill!'

I dashed up to the cockpit and pushed Felix further onto his side. I hauled in the boom, turned *Galatea* into the wind again, clipped my safety harness onto the jackstay, jumped onto the cabin top, leaned against the mast, grabbed the winch handle and rolled the main down, got back into the cockpit and tightened the boom. The wind continued to strengthen, we were pitching from side to side and going off the wind. I turned on the engine, swung the helm hard into the wind to steady her and put her on autohelm.

I leant over Felix. 'Puss, I've sent out the Mayday. They've heard me. They're looking for us. I've taken down the main and the headsail. Puss, please, please, Puss, don't leave me.'

He'd stopped vomiting, but wasn't moving. Dear God, help me!

I couldn't tell if he was conscious. My chest thumped, my temples pounded, but my hands remained steady. I climbed onto the aft cabin top. With legs astride for balance, I took down the mizzen. All the sails were now down. I heard a propeller above me. At last! I saw a red helicopter approach, with a man dangling at the end of a rope. The radio came on and I heard a voice in English: '*Galatea*. We see you, doctor coming.'

The helicopter now hovered above us. The doctor, suspended on a rope, and swinging from side to side, tried to land on deck. *Galatea*'s masts swayed in 90-degree arcs. With legs wide apart on the aft deck, I tried to balance and grab his foot. Twice I touched his toes, twice I lost them. Was this really happening? The wind continued to stiffen, blowing force 5 to 6. *Galatea* wallowed in the rising swell. The doctor spun between the two masts like a trapeze artist. 'Oh God, don't let him get caught in the stays.' The radio came on again: '*Galatea*, this is no good. Too strong wind. We do something...'

I didn't understand the rest. Dear God, don't let them leave me, please don't let them leave me! But they were leaving.

'No!' I screamed when I saw the helicopter move away. Then I heard the faint purr of an engine. I turned. A boat was speeding towards us. Thank goodness! They've called a patrol boat. The helicopter hovered over it, the doctor landed on its deck. The boat sped towards us, and came alongside *Galatea*. I passed them a line. The doctor, slim, barefoot and carrying a rucksack, climbed on board. A heavy, muscular man followed him, took the helm and told me he was the harbour pilot.

'*Merci, merci beaucoup*,' I whispered.

'*Pas de problème.*'

The doctor worked quickly. He raised Felix from his slumped position, pulled equipment out of a plastic box and started a drip.

The pilot switched off the autohelm, revved the engine, put it into gear and motored towards land. I didn't know where he was taking us. Meanwhile, I moved like a zombie, my brain worked like an automaton. I collected Felix's X-rays, medical reports, passports and all the money we had on board.

In the cockpit Felix continued to vomit. The doctor held a bowl under his chin, and gave me a reassuring smile. 'Will be OK, will be OK.'

We approached the wharf.

'*Nous sommes où?* Where are we?' I asked.

'La Grande Motte,' the pilot replied.

We approached the quay and made for the *capitainerie*. A silent crowd was watching. I threw them a line, someone caught it. A stretcher appeared and several men transferred Felix onto it, and took him to a waiting ambulance. He seemed conscious but paralysed on the right side. Suddenly, terror gripped me. They're taking Felix away.

'No, wait!' I shouted and jumped off, rushed towards the ambulance just as the driver turned on the ignition, about to drive off.

'*Non, non, je veux aller avec mon mari!* I want to go with my husband!' I looked into the ambulance. Felix's right arm hung limp. He was conscious, he could see me, but he couldn't speak. The ambulance driver turned to me. '*Je regrette...*' Two paramedics were with Felix, and there was no room for me. I moved back.

'*Quel hôpital allez-vous?* Which hospital are you going to?'

'Guy de Chauliac.' I didn't get it.

'*C'est où?* Where's that?'

He tore off a scrap of newspaper and wrote down the name of the hospital. I grabbed it and read 'Montpellier'.

'*Merci.*'

I moved about like a robot. Two men from the *capitainerie* helped me tie up *Galatea*.

'*Merci beaucoup.*'

'No worries, everything will be OK,' one of them assured me in English. 'We'll look after your boat till you come back.'

I gave them the keys, thanked them again. They called a taxi, I jumped in.

'*C'est l'adresse.*' I gave him the scrap of newspaper.

Now the enormity of what had happened dawned on me. I'd never dealt with our medical problems before. That had always been Felix's department, his decisions. Now I had to face this alone.

'*Combien de temps à Montpellier*? How long to Montpellier?'

'Ah, 40 *minutes.*'

I started to shake uncontrollably. My heart was ready to explode. Only an hour ago, only an hour ago we were celebrating. Was it only an hour ago? What should I do now? Fly Felix to London? I couldn't think clearly. I closed my eyes to calm down, but instead I wept.

Finally, we entered the grounds of a hospital set among palms, flowerbeds, gravel paths and wooden seats. The driver pulled up at the entrance. I read the sign:

Hôpital Neurologique Guy de Chauliac

◎ ◎ ◎ ◎

I still had my safety harness on. I got out, took it off, paid the driver. He had a few words with a young woman waiting at the entrance. She was obviously expecting me. The taxi driver turned and looked at me. His expression was gentle. '*Au revoir, madame, et bonne chance.*' He waved and drove off.

'*Merci,*' I whispered.

I stood there, Felix's medical papers in one hand, the safety harness in the other. In the pockets of my jeans were the passports and money. That was all.

I turned to the young woman, grateful for her kind smile. She took me by the elbow and guided me like a helpless child to an office on the ground floor. Two middle-aged women were sitting at desks. A vase with bright yellow wild flowers relieved the sterility of the room. The women looked up at me as the young woman addressed one of them, but I didn't understand what they were saying. Perhaps this was the local dialect.

Then one of them got up and motioned for me to come with her. I followed her along a long corridor to a lift. Neither of us spoke, but from her dark eyes I sensed that she felt my distress.

It was eerily quiet. The only sound was the monotonous clicking of the woman's heels on the marble floor. My T-shirt was drenched; sweat poured from my forehead. A hot wind swept through windows and down the corridors. The yellow scent of summer drifted in with it.

We entered a small room with a single bed. A nurse was holding Felix's head with one hand, a bowl with the other. The room smelt of vomit. I fell to my knees and gripped his hand to let him know I was with him. 'Honey, I'm here, I'm here…' There was no response.

The nurse looked at me and shook her head slowly. '*Il ne comprends…*' she said. Did she mean that he didn't understand, or did she shake her head because he was so sick?

'*Parlez-vous anglais?* Do you speak English?'

'*Non, je regrette…*' she replied.

Felix's head lay slumped on the pillow, his eyes shut. He'd stopped vomiting, but he looked terrible. I tried again to speak to him. No reply.

A young doctor with honey-coloured hair, china-blue eyes and a friendly smile walked in and extended her hand. '*Je suis Docteur Arlette*.' We shook hands.

She pulled back Felix's sheet and tested his reflexes. She, also, didn't speak English. I gave her Felix's medical papers and struggled to tell her in French that Felix had a history of cancer, radiotherapy, chemotherapy; that all the information was in the notes. Then, without thinking, I asked in English, 'Should I fly him to London? To the Marsden Hospital where he had his original treatment?'

She was horrified. '*Mais c'est pas necessaire.*' Then she added emphatically, '*Absolutement pas necessaire.*'

'In that case I want him to be a private patient,' I struggled in French.

'*Pas necessaire, pas necessaire.* He will have excellent treatment here!'

Confused and sick with worry, I covered my face. 'Dear God, what shall I do?'

Just then two orderlies wheeled a trolley into the room and transferred Felix onto it. The doctor read my face and put an arm round me. '*On le prend pour analyses, radiographie, tout sera bien*, we're taking him for tests, all will be OK,' she assured me.

My legs caved in, I slumped onto a chair. When I'd mustered enough energy, I went down to the office and asked where I could phone my son. '*Mon fils, il est docteur…*he is a doctor in hospital in Sydney.'

'*Bien sûr*, of course, *ici, ici*, here,' the girl said. I gave her David's home number and she dialled for me. David's wife Anne answered. I told her what had happened.

'I'll phone David at the hospital and get him to phone you. Just give me the number.' Some minutes later, David phoned. He was working in the stroke unit at Prince Alfred Hospital in Sydney.

'...I wanted to take Dad to London but they assured me that it's not necessary, that he'll have very good treatment here.'

'I'll find out what people know about the Guy de Chauliac in Montpellier and phone you straight back.' I didn't have to wait long.

'Yes,' he said, 'it's a well known, highly reputable medical centre with excellent facilities. It's perfectly OK to stay there.' I breathed a sigh of relief.

When I returned to the room, Felix still hadn't returned. I looked out the window. On a bench under a palm tree, two people sat and gazed into the distance. It was so quiet. Beds of flowers, shrubs, trees, scent — so beautiful outside, so peaceful, not like my turmoil.

I waited and waited. Why was it taking so long? Had something gone wrong? A nurse brought me a tray with coffee and a sandwich.

'*Merci beaucoup*.' But I couldn't face food.

The sun had set beyond the trees by the time they brought Felix back. His eyes were closed, but some colour had returned to his face. I spoke to him and squeezed his hand. He seemed to recognise my voice, but he couldn't speak.

The young doctor came back to test his reflexes again.

'Do you know the results of the tests?' I asked.

'Non, *le Professeur* will probably come in the morning, he will see the results.'

'Is there a hotel near here where I can stay?'

'If you don't mind sleeping on a stretcher, you can stay with your husband.'

'*Pardon?*' I thought I'd misunderstood. I'd been struggling with French all day. She repeated slowly what she'd said: 'You can sleep on a stretcher next to your husband.'

'*Oh, bien sûr, oui, oui, merci beaucoup.*'

A nurse gave me a hospital gown to sleep in, some torn sheets and pillowcases to use as towels for the shower. 'I am very sorry, but the hospital has no towels. Patients bring their own.'

Relief and gratitude for this kindness overwhelmed me. When I returned from the shower, the stretcher and bedding were already in place. Felix was sound asleep. I kissed him good night and crawled into my bed.

It seemed as if I'd just gone to sleep when the clanking of crockery on a trolley woke me. A cheerful plump woman in green walked in with a tray of croissants on serviettes and coffee in paper cups.

'*Bonjour, madame, bonjour, monsieur. Le petit déjeuner.* Breakfast.'

'*Merci.*' I looked at Felix. He'd opened his eyes, but he looked bewildered and couldn't speak. I reassured him. 'We're in a hospital in Montpellier, honey. I spoke to the kids, and they send their love. David asked about this hospital. It's a big medical centre. There's no need to take you to London. The people are wonderful. They let me sleep in the room with you.

'They did tests and X-rays on you yesterday. The Professor may come today and he'll look at them.'

He nodded, then shut his eyes. I held his hand, dunked a piece of croissant in the coffee and fed him. I put the paper cup to his mouth and he swallowed a few sips. I stroked his brow, his cheeks. I didn't dare leave him.

Doctor Arlette came in several times to see him. I plucked up the courage to ask, 'How is he?'

'He is better, I think, but we will see what the Professor says. Unfortunately, he will not come today. He will come tomorrow, Monday,' she replied.

Every half hour or so nurses dropped in to make sure Felix was comfortable. At first they just smiled, but later they tried to make conversation. I was so grateful for this kindness, the distraction, the relief from tension, from loneliness.

When Felix opened his eyes and I spoke to him, I felt he understood me but couldn't answer. He ate the croissant I fed him and drank the coffee.

The children phoned twice that day. 'Don't worry, Mum, it may take a while for him to start speaking,' David tried to reassure me.

That second night I tossed and turned on the stretcher, and couldn't sleep. A faint morning breeze swept in through the window, relief from the previous day's oppressive heat. I extricated myself from the hospital gown, which had wound itself round me like a straitjacket, and pulled up a chair to Felix's bed. I took his right hand in mine and stroked his head.

From the corridor, a shaft of light lit his face. It was frighteningly grey and furrowed with deep lines around his mouth. I'd never noticed how long and thin his face was, the nose more prominent than ever, the forehead so high. How ill he looked! Unrecognisable. I watched his chest and listened to him breathe.

As I watched over Felix and held his hand, a scene flashed through my mind. How long ago was it — 44 years? Or was it 45?

The school bus. Girls downstairs, boys upstairs. The boys overflowed onto the back platform. I was sitting by myself, behind Vilma and Wanda, two of a select group in my year, girls who attracted boys like bees to honey, who knew how to make even a brown school tunic look sexy. If I'd tried to tighten my belt and hitch up the skirt, I'd have been a laughing stock.

They were sharing a box of Fantales, toffees in yellow wrappers with details of film stars printed all over them. Clark Gable, Tyrone Power, Hedy Lamarr, Katharine Hepburn. Suddenly Vilma turned to Wanda and whispered, 'That's the guy!'

'What guy?'

'You know, the only one who didn't take a girl to the Regatta Dinner.'

Although this information was intended for Wanda, I was close enough to overhear. I was an outsider, and didn't belong to that coterie who went out with boys.

My swift response was to turn and look. He was standing with two others on the back platform. There was no mistaking him. I'd seen his photo in the paper, and knew he was one of the winning eight crew. He had a mop of fair curly hair, small blue eyes and a large nose. Not particularly good-looking. There was nonetheless something attractive about him. A gentleness, perhaps even shyness, not the overbearing bravado one expects of a celebrity member of a winning eight.

He wasn't talking to anyone. I looked at him closely and wondered why he hadn't asked anyone to the school year's most prestigious event, the Regatta Dinner. I liked his round face. He was not in uniform. Uniform was only compulsory for girls. He wore a brown jacket and pale green trousers. I couldn't believe the trousers. Pale green! I hated green.

Felix stirred and opened his eyes. I smiled and squeezed his hand, then bent over and kissed him. 'How are you, sweetheart?' He nodded with his eyes. There was a faint smile.

'Do you know what I've been reminiscing about? The bus, that school special. Remember? Do you know how long ago that was? Was it 44 or 45 years? Remember those terrible green pants of yours? And how I never got over the fact that I could have gone to that Regatta Dinner if only we'd met two weeks earlier and you'd asked me?'

He smiled. He wanted to say something but couldn't.

'Remember how we both got to the bus stop earlier and earlier each day? It took you three days to say "hello" and I felt myself go red from the neck up, like a rash. And then when you asked me to go dinghy sailing, I couldn't very well tell you that I couldn't swim more than 25 yards without drowning. I didn't have a choice, did I? I was 15 and had never been out with a boy. And remember how I killed myself laughing when I found out that your nickname at the Scouts was "Puss" because of "Felix the Cat", and that stayed with you forever?'

Felix looked at me, his eyes moist.

'And look at us now,' I said sniffing. 'My one and only boyfriend, and we're on a boat in France. Just temporarily in hospital.'

My spirits rose when I saw Felix that morning. He had more colour, he hadn't vomited for almost 24 hours and, although he still couldn't speak, he wasn't distressed. The nurses continued to come in frequently to check on him. He started to drink by himself, holding the cup with one hand.

As I calmed down, my French improved and I had no problems communicating.

An Australian we'd met some weeks earlier drove the long way from Castelnaudary to Montpellier when I contacted him. He, too, reassured me that Felix would be well looked after at this hospital. When I mentioned that one of the nurses had offered to take me shopping, he volunteered to drive me to La Grande Motte to pick up the clothes and toiletries Felix and I needed.

We found *Galatea* tied up under the *capitainerie* window, still in everyone's way, but as the staff had promised, they were looking after her. On the way back from La Grande Motte, we picked up a Montpellier paper, in which a short article appeared:

MALAISE CARDIAQUE A BORD
D'UN VOILIER AUSTRALIEN

Avant 15 h. hier, un pneumatique de la Société nationale de sauvetage mer a secouru un couple d'Australiens en détresse, à 9 km, au large de Palavas...

HEART ATTACK ON BOARD
AN AUSTRALIAN SAILING VESSEL

Just before 3 pm, a coastal patrol rescue boat came to the aid of an Australian couple in distress, 9 km off Palavas...

When *le Professeur* — a tall, impressive, sombre man — visited Felix on the Monday, he assured me that the tests didn't indicate a severe stroke. 'But it is hard to tell how quick or how complete the recovery will be.' He always spoke French and let me struggle, although I suspected that he spoke English.

The weather continued to be excruciatingly hot, especially in our tiny room.

'*Il fait très, très chaud ici. La chaleur est terrible.* The heat is terrible,' said Claudette, the nurse-in-charge, on the third morning. 'I think we'll move you to a bigger room, which is cooler,' she added. They brought in a wheelchair for Felix and I pushed him into our new room. 'Hey, two proper beds,' I said triumphantly, 'and the room is bigger than most hotel rooms!'

Felix smiled and, in a slurred speech I could barely decipher, said, 'Could've made it a double bed.' He was awake most of the time now, more active and interested in his surroundings. He started to put down his legs several times a day, then tried to take a few steps leaning on me. Some days later, we walked along the corridor.

'Hey, Puss, you're doing great guns. You're going further each time. Maybe tomorrow or the day after we could go down in the lift and walk in the garden.'

From the windows of our room, we watched with proprietorial affection as each day the red Pompiers helicopter belonging to the fire brigade flew into the grounds of the hospital with medical emergencies. Sometimes, in an exuberant mood, I hung out the window, waved and blew them kisses.

The nursing staff, Doctor Arlette, Felix and I established a jovial relationship. This was the summer holiday season, the hospital was not full and the staff not overworked, so they used any excuse to come in and chat. A constant stream of visitors came in and out of our room. Felix and I had rarity value. We were Australian and spoke peculiar French. All of us laughed and joked at our attempts to communicate in French and English. Our French was more daring by the day and reached a stage where we could talk about our lives.

These nurses, like so many other women we met during the months we spent in France, often asked, 'What's it like in Australia? Do the men help at home?' Invariably they complained, '...all of us work, but the men still expect us to do everything — go to work, look after the home and the children. They don't lift a finger, and even expect hot meals at lunchtime if they come home...'

Many of them were pieds-noirs, French Algerians like our neighbours on the marina in Sète, and lived a long way from the hospital. Some drove several hours to and from work each day.

'We have to live where we can afford to buy a house, and a lot depends on where our husbands find work. It's not easy.'

As the days progressed, my mood veered from terrible distress to an unreasonable euphoria. I started to write mad letters home, behaving as if it had all been a big joke.

'Honey, better not post this letter, it'll confuse them, it wasn't that funny. Wait a while...' Felix realised that I was not entirely rational, and in his calm way tried to tone me down.

The little shop on the ground floor became my corner grocery. When I visited it each morning to buy the paper, fruit and biscuits, I also had to report to Madame Dupré.

'*Alors*,' she'd start. '*Comment ça va aujourd'hui?* How are things today?'

'Oh! *La, la!*' She exclaimed the first time I took Felix down past the shop into the garden. She clapped her hands and beamed.

When David phoned each day, I told him what investigations were being done. '...And he's having such difficulty walking. I hold him up but he can only go up and down the corridor twice, then he's exhausted.'

'Mum, I can assure you he's having exactly the same tests and the same treatment in Montpellier that he'd be having here in Sydney. It'll take time, you've got to be patient.'

A small, middle-aged Vietnamese doctor, with a round face and kind eyes, visited frequently. He always sat on Felix's bed, held his hand and spoke slowly to make sure we understood. '*Tout sera bien*, all will be OK,' he assured us. His manner was gentle and concerned, as if we were part of his family.

The day before Felix was discharged, *le Professeur* came on a round with his minions. 'Under no circumstances are you to climb up the mast,' he said, in French, of course.

'*Pas de problème!*' Felix assured him. '*Ma femme le fait.* My wife will do that.'

'Like bloody hell I'll go up the mast!'

Felix winked. I wanted to cry out with joy. My old Felix winked.

'And you come and see me in six weeks,' *le Professeur* added.

On the morning of our departure, Felix managed to have a shower with minimum help from me, but I had to help him dress. Then I gathered our few belongings into a plastic bag and we were ready.

Doctor Arlette and the three nurses we had come to know so well wished us *bon voyage*. '*Au revoir, et bonne chance!*'

We were so pleased to know that we'd see them again when we returned for a check-up with *le Professeur* in six weeks.

During the two weeks we'd spent at the Guy de Chauliac, I had grown to love the place and also to appreciate the kindness that went beyond anything I'd expected from a hospital. I didn't feel alone, I felt at home there. Our bilingual efforts made us all laugh. I loved the garden with its scents and splashes of summer flowers. I can still feel the warm benches where I sat under swaying palms, the warm breeze and the gravel paths under my feet. I can still hear the sound of the red helicopter's rotors, the voice of Claudette, '*Ah, mon dieu, la chaleur, la chaleur.*'

We waved until we were out of the gates and out of sight. With tears running down my cheeks, I gave Felix a hug. He'd lost weight and felt thin. Thank God, we'd survived. We held hands as we had after his first radiotherapy treatment in London.

'We were lucky to be off the coast of France when all this happened, so lucky. And we've learnt so much about the kindness of strangers,' I said.

'Yes,' Felix replied. He squeezed my hand, tears in his eyes.

chapter three

'We're back!' I gave Felix a bear hug as I helped him step into the sunshine of La Grande Motte. He was again close to tears. We stood motionless next to the taxi and looked at our *Galatea* tied up in everyone's way, just as I'd left her two weeks earlier.

Yachties coming in to the *capitainerie* fastened to her starboard and stepped across her deck to get ashore. After the tranquillity of the hospital, we were no longer used to the loud music and noise that bombarded us. Like Cap d'Agde, this was a *port de plaisance*, a busy, restless resort in mid-summer.

Captain Alain, who was in charge of the *capitainerie*, waved from his upstairs window. A small man with greying hair, he had a shy, reserved manner. Georges, his assistant, a sturdy man with a gentle touch, helped Felix over *Galatea*'s rails and into the cockpit. I made for the gangway, opened the hatches and let the breeze sweep through, but Felix looked frail and bewildered by the commotion.

'Just sit here for a while, sweetie, don't rush…' I sat down with him and put my arm around him. 'I know it's hard to believe, but we're back, and you'll be OK. Everyone said you would be, but it'll take time.'

It was mid-morning and the sun beat down through the Mediterranean haze.

'What a good thing we have a permanent awning,' I said. Felix just nodded.

A crowd of holiday-makers with hats and bags stood on the quay and watched boats sail in and out of the harbour, children chased one another, flags fluttered, horns honked and the air smelt of sea and salt and summer.

'It's so good to be back on board,' Felix whispered as if talking to himself. 'Back home.' He looked insecure and tired, but his face had shed much of its earlier greyness.

'Yes, it is,' I replied. 'Hey, how about the luxury of sleeping on feather pillows tonight, and soft blankets and thick towels? Five-star luxury.'

We continued to sit in silence in the cockpit and watch the passing parade.

'I think I'll go down now,' Felix said after a while.

'Isn't it great to have rails everywhere, so you can hang on, inside and outside?'

'Even though they weren't quite meant for post-stroke recuperating yachties.'

'But they'll come in useful,' I said.

I helped him down to the saloon. He looked around as if to convince himself that we really were back. While he rested, I stacked away the food I'd bought on the way back from Montpellier. The cheeses, salamis, sausages, pâtés, stuffed artichokes, green olives stuffed with pimentos, black olives stuffed with anchovies, yoghurts...all went into the fridge with the *tarte tatin* at the top. Then I put clean sheets on our bunk, aired the pillows and blankets and hosed down the deck.

Felix ate very little. He seemed more withdrawn than he'd been during the last days at the hospital. At night we clung to each other in our double bunk. My mood alternated between relief and concern. I wondered what was going through his mind. I tossed in bed and thought about how he'd always protected me, rarely burdening me with worries if he could avoid it. Now we faced a reversal. My new role was to look after him, to protect him. But when the problems were medical, how could I? He knew more than I what our future had in store for us, what we should do. But at the time neither of us wanted to talk about it.

He was asleep now, still clinging to my hand. I loved the photos of Emma and Jackie on the bulkhead. I wished they were here, or we were nearer home. Oh, the heat. It was so oppressive, the ceiling so low, the space so confined. The thumping music was pounding my temples. Perhaps one of the basils in the cockpit hadn't died, I loved that scent. I'd check tomorrow. Reminded me of our garden at home. But it was no longer our garden or our home. I wondered how it looked. My stomach was churning like a dishwasher. I tasted the nougat chocolate. Shouldn't have had the pork pâté. We were rocking, the water was slapping against the quay, the fenders slipping up and down. If only I could sleep! Puss was stirring. I was so relieved when I felt him move.

If he didn't see us on deck by 9, Georges invariably came to check that we were all right. After a few days we'd established a routine. My first port of call each morning was the *boulanger* for a baguette. By now we wouldn't dream of eating a morning baguette in the evening. After breakfast, I helped Felix ashore — first one leg over the rail, then the other — and supported him while we staggered along for his morning constitutional. On the first day, we didn't go far. After that a little further each time. Some days he needed more propping up than others. Often, along the way, we rested on seats and watched the passing parade.

'This is such a different crowd from the Riviera. No glamour here,' I said. '*Ports de plaisance* are where the "ordinary" French go on vacation. More flats than hotels. More interesting to observe than the Riviera.'

'For more observation I think it's time for us to go to the *pâtisserie* and then check out the *charcuterie* next door,' Felix said. I felt like hugging him when he came out with these Felixisms.

'Of course. The focal point of our day.'

What La Grande Motte lacked in the romance of the old fishing port of Sète, it made up in food shops. The window display of our favourite *pâtisserie* was mesmerising. It was no easy matter to decide which *gâteau* to test each day.

'Choices, choices, choices…' Felix said.

Meringues filled with whipped cream and topped with berries soaked in Grand Marnier, scooped oranges filled with *crème pâtissière* or confectioner's custard topped with caramel chips, meringue with chestnut cream topped with chantilly, orange cake with mocca icing, caramel logs filled with dark nougat, profiteroles with chocolate sauce, berry tartlets…The range was endless. Sometimes we settled for parfaits, or a sorbet ice to go with iced coffee or iced tea or iced mocca, or a fruit granita. The decorations were extravaganzas in sculptured fantasies and designs.

'You must try the *tulip framboise*. It is tulip pastry with raspberry sherbet and fresh raspberry sauce, it is beautiful. And on top are fresh red currants,' our friendly helpers behind the counter advised us.

'We did not see you yesterday. We think that you have left us!'

'*Mais, non! C'est impossible!*' I answered. A visit to the *pâtisserie* or the *charcuterie* never failed to cheer Felix. Diet was not something we worried about. 'Everything in moderation, ho ho,' Felix said.

To brighten the saloon, I filled vases with flowers and replaced the geraniums, the basil and the mint, which hadn't survived our absence. We loved to brush the basil and sniff the burst of scent that filled the cockpit and drifted into the saloon.

But the euphoria that had gripped me in the hospital when I knew Felix had survived soon dissipated. Although his walking improved each day, his eyes had become the new problem. No matter how hard he tried, he couldn't read until the afternoon.

'My eyes feel as if they're rotating. They don't stop moving, I can't focus.' Tears of frustration rolled down his cheeks. He was so depressed, it broke me up. When I couldn't bear to see him like this, I made excuses to go ashore. 'I think I should take the wash to the laundrette. I'll be back as soon as I can, honey.' By the time I got back he was usually asleep.

Sometimes I told him I was going to the hairdresser, but in fact I sat on a bench, wrote letters, wept or phoned the kids from a booth. Much of the time I watched couples chatting, with arms around each other, children skipping or tossing balls, parents pushing strollers. Everywhere there was sound and movement, loud music and the smell of coffee. Once, an old woman with elephantine legs and heavy shopping bags noticed me cry. She stopped and gave me a sad, sympathetic smile. Some days later she passed again and gave me a broad smile. Her '*Bonjour, madame, quelle belle journée*, what a beautiful day' made me feel good.

'What should I do? Where do we go from here?' I kept asking myself. In the hospital I was ecstatic, relieved that Felix was getting better, that he was in an excellent hospital, that he could speak again, that his walking gradually improved. Here, I missed the doctors' reassurance, the nurses' banter. I felt alone.

Felix hadn't noticed that in one week I'd told him I was going to the hairdresser three times. He hadn't noticed that my hair looked no different.

◎◎◎◎

July, August. The heat glowed and sat on us. Transparent and iridescent, it rose from concrete pavements and asphalt like ghosts drifting up from hell. Day after day, not a breath blew through *Galatea*. With four fans blowing and wet tea towels suspended from the hand rails and over our faces, we lay on our bunks in swimsuits to get cool.

'Honey, if the worst of your migraine is over, perhaps we could go out and get some air. It's after 10. Should be much cooler now,' Felix suggested one evening.

'I can't stand flashing lights, and you know I never exhibit myself outside in a bikini.'

'Oh, come on. Put on your big straw sun hat, keep your eyes closed and put on your darkest sunglasses.'

'I'll look like a lunatic. At night, in a hat and sunglasses.'

'What the hell,' he said. Yes, I thought, what the hell!

And so we tottered into the bright night lights — Felix in a swimsuit, barefoot and unsteady, hanging on to me, barefoot in a bikini with a large sun hat, sunglasses and eyes shut.

'Puss, don't lean so heavily on me, I can't hold you up. I'm fragile!'

'I'll try.' We staggered on.

'Careful now. Coming to an uneven bit and a step after that,' he warned me. I shuffled forward.

'What if someone from Sydney sees us?' The thought suddenly struck me.

'They wouldn't recognise us.'

'What if a policeman notices us?'

'We'll tell him we're Australians, that'll explain everything. Come on, there's a bench over here, let's sit down.' Clasping my hand, he guided me towards it. I curled my fingers in his hand, a broad, square hand with short, stubby fingers. Smooth, warm, gentle, secure.

'We're going great guns with one pair of eyes and one pair of steady legs!' he said reassuringly. 'Ah, the breeze! Can you feel that breeze?'

I felt the breeze. But the flashing neon lights penetrated my sunhat, sunglasses, eyelids. Zigzag, technicolour fireworks. Loud music beat on my right hemisphere. Boom, boom, boom.

'What a relief, thank God for this breeze.' I heaved a sigh. 'If only we could get away from the heat for a few hours a day. What do you think about picking up the car and going on small drives?'

'It's OK by me, but I know you don't like driving a manual, or driving on the right. But if you're prepared to drive, we could get a taxi to Sète tomorrow.'

'I'll give it a go if you act as back-seat driver.'

It seemed an eternity since we'd left our car with Madame Thomas for a service.

'*C'est pas de problème*, no problem, wait till your husband is OK,' she'd said when I phoned from Montpellier to tell her that I didn't know when we'd pick it up.

My hands trembled as I slipped into the driver's seat and clicked the seat belt shut. Felix rested his hand on my lap. 'You'll be OK, just relax.'

I turned on the ignition. Crrrrunch! I turned it off.

'Start again, honey. Put your foot on the clutch, turn on the ignition, then put the gear handle into reverse and lift the clutch very slowly while you put your foot on the gas.'

I put my foot on the clutch, shifted the gear handle into reverse, turned on the ignition then put on the gas. The car went into a spasm of hiccups.

'I'll break the gearbox!' I was close to tears. A trickle of sweat ran down my chest. I didn't want to drive.

'Let me take her out, then you can start on the road. But if you don't want to drive, we can leave the car here until I can drive.'

'No, it's OK, I hate it, but I'll get used to it,' I mumbled.

We changed seats, and Felix backed out of the garage. Madame Thomas's wrinkled face beamed benevolently. She'd refused to charge us the four weeks' garaging and gave us a bag of plums from her garden.

'*Bonne chance, et bon voyage*,' she waved.

Driving at snail's pace, we made it to the old Sète marina. A small work boat now occupied the spot where we'd been. Giselle and Francis's boat was gone. The flower vendors on the quay were gathering buckets of flowers and folding their stalls at the end of their day, the supermarket had already closed for lunch and siesta, and the street was deserted. The restaurant awnings were down, but few tables were occupied. Window shutters facing the water were closed to darken rooms and keep out the midday sun. A fisherman, rope in hand, stood at the bow of an incoming boat, ready to tie it to a bollard. Seagulls circled in tow.

My heart missed a beat as we entered the yacht club's dining room. It was almost full and, as always, mostly with men. The whole room turned to look and greet us although we recognised only a few faces. They must have read about us in the paper. In a place like this news spread fast. They noticed Felix's insecure walk and my protective arm around him and soon turned their gaze back to their plates. The hum of conversation continued. We wished them '*bon appétit*'.

The waiter rushed to clear a table near the window and pulled out a chair.

'*Alors, comment ça va?*'

'*Assez bien*, we're OK. How are you? Where are Giselle and Francis?'

'They left a few days ago, somewhere further along the coast to a new job.'

'*Quel dommage*, what a pity, we'd hoped to see them.'

The dazzling hors d'oeuvres on the buffet table smelt delicious. Grilled eggplant, stuffed tomatoes, olives, tuna, jellied egg, sausage. I felt a bout of nostalgia as we gazed down on the marina where, only weeks earlier, we'd started on our adventure with such enthusiasm and optimism. The familiar smell of Languedoc cuisine drifted in from the kitchen. Subdued, we ate in silence while we looked at the scavenging seagulls and the fishing boats below.

Four weeks. Nothing had changed outside. But we...

I parked the car next to the *capitainerie* and switched off the ignition. My shirt was soaked. I didn't move, waited for the flutter in my stomach to subside. Felix put his arm around me.

'You were great! Not even a near collision.' He laughed. It was good to see him laugh. A black cat marched past me. I bent to pat her for good luck. She turned, looked at me with disdain and trotted off purposefully to a rendezvous.

As we stepped on board, I swiped the basil. It did its trick and released a wave of scent. The geranium had sprouted three bright red blooms in the past two days. Our plants were happy. I opened the hatches to let a draft through, popped my head out and waved to Georges, who stood at the upstairs window of the *capitainerie*. He beamed, pointed to our car and made a 'vee for victory' sign. Felix put on Pavarotti, Carreras and Domingo full volume to drown out the noise outside.

'Come back to Sorrento,' they sang *à trois*.

'Wait till we get there, kid. Wait till we get there!'

Felix was cheerful. For the first time he could get up the stairs to the *capitainerie* showers for an unrationed supply of hot water.

'Don't forget the number you must press on the keypad to get in,' Georges had called out to him. 'Yes, I've written it down,' Felix assured him.

'I'll have a shower too, and then wait for you here at the top of the stairs,' I said.

There were two showers in the women's bathroom — A and B. It was after 6, the time to get ready *pour la promenade et le dîner.* There were four ahead of me, and we waited patiently. Suddenly the entrance door buzzed open, and in rushed an almost nude young man with a miniscule towel wrapped carelessly round his waist. Stunned by this apparition, I blurted 'Hello? Hello?' whereupon he gave me a broad smile and flew past to knock on shower door A, exclaiming, '*C'est toi, Monique?*' The response was instant, loud and clear: '*Oui, chéri, entres...*come in!'

Others in the queue didn't react to the mirth and giggles in cubicle A. But I felt more Anglo than I had ever felt. When I'd previously had a shower in cubicle A, I'd noticed a full-length mirror with two of its corner hinges missing. There was no bench or screen to keep a towel or clothes dry, and when I bent to pick up my towel from the floor, I almost knocked off that mirror. How French! Just a full-length mirror! How many people would want to look at themselves in a steamy full-length mirror? I had visions of Monique and her *chéri* banging on the mirror, followed by a loud crash and splinters of glass everywhere.

Meanwhile, three people had been in and out of the other shower, and there was still no sign of an end to the shenanigans in cubicle A. When I'd had my shower and came out of cubicle

B, they were still frolicking, and I couldn't wait for the crash. As I went out, I saw Felix emerge from the men's showers.

'Guess what goes on in the men's showers?' he said.

'Not in the men's showers too?'

'There's no end to the things we're learning about French culture!'

When I returned from the baker with our breakfast baguette the following morning, Felix looked close to tears. Stooped over the navigation table, his brow furrowed, a tremor in his hands, he sat trying to focus on a book propped in front of him. Mornings were always bad, no matter how hard he tried.

'Puss, don't try so hard. Your eyes will take time to go back to normal.'

'No! I must go on trying, otherwise we won't get anywhere.'

'They told you at the hospital that it may take months for things to get back to normal.' I tried to console him, gave him a hug, then added, 'I'll make coffee, and we'll have breakfast outside. Bacon and eggs. I can smell the bacon and hear the sizzle even before I've taken them out of the fridge.' He didn't hear, wasn't listening.

'What if it has nothing to do with the stroke — if it's lymphoma, another recurrence?'

The shock stopped me in my tracks. I didn't know what to say. 'If that's what you're thinking, Puss, then we'd better fly to London.'

He thought for a while, then replied, 'I guess so. If it's not a recurrence, there'll be no treatment, and we'll be back in a few days. I'll get used to the eyes, and hope they'll improve.' After a long pause, he added, 'There's not much chance of getting to Corsica or Sardinia this year, but we could sail a short way along the coast if the Professor in Montpellier says it's OK to go. You can read the charts, you're the navigator.'

'Yes, that's a good idea,' I tried to sound enthusiastic. 'We can phone London after breakfast, and see what they say.'

We were deep in thought as we walked to the Telecom office. I tried not to think about our future. Sometimes I wondered whether Felix did. He was pushing himself so hard and I couldn't bear to watch it. The girl at the telephone exchange knew us well by now, and treated us like favoured customers. With bright red lips, short, curly dark hair and lively green eyes, she had a dazzling array of clothes that looked as if they'd come from Aladdin's cave.

'*Alors*, calling Australia again?' she asked. 'It is such fun to hear the telephone ring in Australia.'

'No, it's London this time.' Felix gave her the number.

'Oh!' she laughed, pretending to be disappointed.

'*Numéro cinq.*'

We walked to booth 5. Felix picked up the receiver, smiled reassuringly at me and squeezed my hand. I heard the ring at the other end. I looked at Felix. He was composed, with no visible trace of nervousness. 'Hello, I'm calling from France, can you put me through to Dr Hunt please?…I see, well then can I speak to his offsider…thank you.'

I walked away, my heart pounding. I waited, I didn't want to hear the conversation, then I turned back. Felix was nodding into the receiver. 'Yes, all right then, I'll book a flight for next Wednesday, and I'll see Dr Hunt at 9 o'clock on Thursday… thank you very much.'

He hung up the phone and walked towards me. I was struck by the dark rings round his eyes, his lined face. How much he'd aged in the past weeks!

'What did they say?'

'Most people are still on holidays. Mike Hunt will be back next week, so we'll need to book a flight for Wednesday. His offsider doesn't think it's likely to be lymphoma, but you can never tell, and he agrees that it ought to be checked. So that's it, we'll need to get ourselves organised to leave in a week!'

As we walked back, I wondered — what complications next? Radiotherapy, chemotherapy, stroke, now the eyes...

Felix looked at me, noticed my concern. 'Sweetie, don't look so upset, this may be nothing. In any case, you know us. We do whatever we can to solve our problems. Then we live around them and get on with life as best we can.'

'You're right, Puss. Meanwhile, we have a few days up our sleeves. How about we drive to Aigues-Mortes tomorrow. There are lots of interesting places not far from here.'

'That's a good idea,' he said, but he sounded so tired. I knew we had to do something to get away from the excruciating heat of the marina and *Galatea*, especially as people were walking on and off our deck all day long to get to the *capitainerie*. I wasn't happy driving, but I had to. And so, for the following days we went on excursions.

Aigues-Mortes, a few kilometres inland from La Grande Motte, is an ancient town built 700 years ago by Saint Louis as a base for his crusade to Jerusalem. Its massive stone ramparts and walls, towers and gates had once been surrounded by a moat, now filled and used as a car park. As we parked, the walls of the town glowed dull gold. We walked through a gate into a quiet, stone world. Patterns of light and shade danced along the meandering lanes and alleys. Ornate pots of geraniums flanked front doors. But the place was deserted. It was lunchtime, and the heat was stifling. Even the two restaurants we passed were almost empty. We were there because this was the time of day when Felix's eyes felt better, when they irritated him less. He was, however, too tired to continue walking.

'Let's go into that restaurant, it has a couple of fans,' he said. We had a salad, cold *vin de la maison*, and rested. After a while it was still too hot to go sightseeing so we decided to go home. On the way back to La Grande Motte we stopped to book the flight from Montpellier to London.

'We'll be back within a week and spend the rest of the summer sailing along the coast to Marseilles and the Iles d'Hyères, Pomègues and Cassis, and then we'll go on trips inland...' Felix tried hard to reassure me.

When Georges came on board to have a drink with us, we told him our latest woes. 'We'll be going to London for tests to find out what the problem is with my eyes,' Felix said. 'If I need treatment, we could be away for four to six weeks. If I don't, then we'll be back within a week. We're wondering where we could leave *Galatea*.'

'That's no problem,' Georges assured us. 'You leave her right here and we'll look after her, like we did before. I'm sure the Captain will agree.'

'You are all so wonderful! We don't know how we can ever thank you, but this time what should we do with the car? Is there a garage near here?'

'Under the window on the other side over there,' he pointed to the side of the *capitainerie*.

'But that has a big "No Parking" sign.'

'Don't worry, you will have no problem, we will arrange it.'

We couldn't believe our luck.

'Where shall we stay in London?' I asked Felix as we stepped on board.

'I'm sure we can stay with friends for a few days. But if we have to stay for several weeks, then we'll have to rent a place.'

'It's OK for us to rent a place each year for the winter months, but if we have to return to London unexpectedly, we'll have to get a tiny pad. A place where we can stay at any time,' I said.

'We'll see.'

◎ ◎ ◎ ◎

We were subdued when we arrived in London. For several months now, we hadn't seen friends or spoken English without mentally translating into French. The few English friends we had were away on holidays, but three Australian couples, all old friends, were visiting London at the time. Finding them there was a breath of home. They gave us the support we badly needed at a time when we were both close to the edge of what we could endure.

London Underground in August, the crush of people, sweaty bodies making for the summer sales, unconditioned air; we were no longer used to a city atmosphere.

The first time we'd gone along this route to the hospital, the trees had been autumnal, the lawns a carpet of golden leaves. Now this well trodden path along Sumner Place and Onslow Square was in the grip of high summer. Cinerarias, petunias, phlox and pelargoniums spilled over window boxes. Tubs of azaleas, cumquats and daisy bushes flanked front doors. In the midst of traffic turmoil, some chose to sunbake in the squares. This was summer in London.

When we reached the entrance to the Marsden, we felt like old customers. We made for our usual corner seats next to a coffee table piled high with old magazines. Even where one chooses to sit can become a habit.

'Dr Huber, Dr Hunt will see you now.'

'Well, so what's been happening?'

As Felix started to tell Dr Hunt the story of the stroke, the rescue and Montpellier Hospital, I switched off. Dr Hunt listened, and finally said, 'Well, Felix, it doesn't sound to me as if it's going to have anything to do with lymphoma, but we can't exclude it. We've all had our surprises. I'd like some X-rays, blood tests, an MRI. I think it'd also be a good idea for you to see an ophthalmologist. When you've had all these tests done, I'd like to see you again, and we'll take it from there.'

For four days Felix had an endless array of blood tests, X-rays and an MRI. Two days later, we had another appointment with Dr Hunt to discuss the final results. Felix was composed, but I knew from the slight tremor of his lip that he was nervous.

'You may come in now, Dr Huber,' the nurse said.

We followed her. The door to the consulting room was open. I saw Dr Hunt's face. He was smiling broadly. 'Thank God,' I said under my breath as we walked in. 'Thank God,' I turned to Felix, and both of us beamed.

The next day the ophthalmologist confirmed that the eyes were rotating.

'This happens with strokes sometimes. It takes time, but eventually it will improve. It's a great nuisance, but it's nothing to worry about.'

We were exuberant as we stepped out of the taxi at the airport.

'I think people are looking at us as if we're nuts or on our honeymoon.'

We had one suitcase between us. Was that a dare that all would be well, that we'd be back on *Galatea* within one week, although we had been prepared for six weeks of radiotherapy?

'It's all clear, Puss!' I squeezed Felix's arm and wanted to shout to the world that life was beautiful.

We stood in a long queue to luggage control. We worked our way through passport and customs, then ambled into the passenger lounge. We had a lot of time.

'Let's look for the fanciest breakfast place.'

'Over there,' Felix suggested. 'The one with that kitsch.' Posters of green Swiss meadows with satisfied Nestlé cows grazing among alpine flora, balloons in a blue sky and children walking hand in hand along a vanishing path hung on the walls.

'Muesli! They must have muesli here!' I was ecstatic. I smelt coffee, bacon and eggs, and said, 'Look, Danish pastries.'

After breakfast Felix spotted a chocolate shop. 'Swiss chocolates. Just what we need on *Galatea*!' We beamed as we walked in. Felix made for the counter while I went to the other side and admired a merry-go-round made of chocolate animals. As I looked up over the display, I saw a face staring at me from a vast wall mirror. Was that me? I shuddered. Owl rings around the eyes. A haggard face in need of sleep. Hair in need of a cut. Was this really me? I turned away, my heart raced. Meanwhile, Felix's eyes were locked onto trays of chocolates in every shape along the counter. I saw a girl with impeccable looks behind it, waiting for Felix to make his selection. I heard her answer Felix's questions.

'This one, sir? This is crunchy nougatine and dark chocolate, this one is marzipan.'

'I'd like four of each of these please.'

A young couple walked in and admired the merry-go-round. The woman was casually dressed in a light grey suit and a pink blouse. She carried a leather handbag that matched her expensive shoes. Sunglasses sat on her dark, shiny hair. She pointed with manicured nails and Georg Jensen rings to the chocolate merry-go-round.

'*Ist das nicht süss?* Isn't that cute?' She was enchanted. I wanted to run away, to hide in my faded-from-washing jeans and shapeless T-shirt, toting my antique model overnight bag and computer. What was wrong with me? I was being oversensitive. Only minutes earlier I'd been deliriously happy. Now I wanted to disappear. I was jealous! That wasn't like me. What was happening to me?

At last, thank God, the girl was wrapping the box in gold paper and a red bow. Felix looked delighted with himself. I went outside to check the flight board.

'Come on Puss, we're boarding, Gate 5.'

He locked his arm into mine. I started to cry.

The plane took off. 'Why am I so edgy?' I wondered. 'Why did I lose my cool in the chocolate shop? Pull yourself together, kid,' I said to myself. 'Felix is all clear. Think of sailing the South of France. All you need is a haircut, a tint, a new T-shirt, a pair of sandals. Sit in the sun, get some colour.'

We boarded the plane. I looked at Felix. He looked so happy.

'I think this is the time to get stuck into the chocolates,' he said as he started to untie the red bow on the chocolate box the girl had spent half an hour getting right.

'A drink, madam, sir?' the cabin stewardess asked. Well, at least this Air France stewardess looked normal. She had a few spots on her face and her hair hadn't been done since she'd left Paris that morning.

'Nothing for me, thanks,' I answered.

'I'll have a whisky with a lot of soda.'

'Chocolates and whisky don't go.' My tone was abrupt.

'I'll try it and tell you.'

'Can you eat lunch?' I asked Felix.

'You bet.'

I hadn't seen him eat so much for weeks.

'Puss, do you remember when we were in our teens and every Sunday night we had twelve eggs, three frankfurters cut in, and a tin of peaches? Scrambled eggs was the only thing I could cook!'

'How could I forget?' He smiled.

The plane was full of people going on holidays to the South of France. They'd read *A Year in Provence*, and were in search of a dream. We were in search of our dream too. On *Galatea*. But oh, I was tired. Oh, so tired. Exhausted. Of course I wanted to move on. But sometimes I wished I could spend one week in a hospital bed. Just sleeping.

Felix was full of *joie de vivre* now, and it was so good to see him like this. He still couldn't read in the morning but it seemed to worry him less. Since he'd had the OK, he'd been on such a high. He must have been really worried.

'I bought some cards for Emma and Jackie. The Guards changing at Buckingham Palace, Horse Guards, Tower of London. Here, you write them one and I'll write them one,' I suggested.

I gave him a card and a pen. He balanced it on a magazine, wrote the date, then stopped. Said nothing. Then: 'I can't write. I'll type them a letter on the computer when we get on *Galatea* tonight.' I turned and looked at him. His mood had changed.

'What's wrong?'

'I can't control the pen. It slides across.'

I took a deep breath. 'Don't worry, I'll write for you, you just sign.'

'No, I don't feel like it.'

'OK, let's not write anything. Which chocolate is the praline? I feel like a praline.'

But it was too late. His exuberant mood had vanished. We looked out the window. High above, a thick layer of grey–white and pink clouds drifted past. The sky was a faint purple, the setting sun a mango gold.

'Ladies and gentlemen, we're about to start our descent. Please fasten your seat belts!'

We fastened our belts and locked fingers.

Our mood was still subdued as the buildings of La Grande Motte loomed closer. We stepped out of the taxi. *Galatea* and our Renault were exactly where we'd left them. The quay buzzed with traffic and activity at the end of the day. Holiday-makers in boats were arriving back in port, children were jumping, calling out, women clutching shopping bags stepped back on board. Loud music. Georges, busy with incoming yachts, looked surprised and pleased to see us.

'Ah, welcome back! I hope this is good news. We thought you would be away many weeks.'

'It's good news. You'll be rid of us soon and we'll be out of everyone's way!'

'It's very good for you. I have letters for you. I'll bring them down when I finish here.'

'Thank you, Georges. It's good to be back.'

We climbed on board past people clambering on and off our deck. Of our plants, only the red geranium had survived. The rest had died of thirst. We opened the hatches and climbed down into the saloon. It looked tidy, unlived in. No newspaper or open books on the table, no flowers, no hat thrust onto a bunk, no half-filled glasses at the sink.

'Won't take long and we'll be back in business,' Felix said.

'God, I'm suffering from tartlet deprivation. Puss, would you mind going ashore and getting a baguette and milk and fruit and tartlets, and maybe some *charcuterie*, while I unpack. I'll hose down the cockpit too. You might as well take the pot plants and bury them in the rubbish bins. We'll get new ones tomorrow.'

'OK. I shouldn't be too long.'

'Here is your mail,' Georges said as he passed down a bundle of letters. Fat letters with Australian stamps. A wave of homesickness gripped me. I undid the string and opened the top envelope. It was from a friend. I read quickly, down the page:

> …we're so sorry to hear that Felix still has problems with his eyes and that you're thinking of going to London to get it checked up. Perhaps the sensible thing would be to do something other than take risks sailing…

I didn't want to read on. But I couldn't stop. I swallowed the temptation to cry. Yes, maybe it'd be sensible, but that wasn't what Felix wanted to do. And nor did I. His confidence would be shattered if we had to stop sailing. I knew that. He needed to build up his confidence. And if taking risks was what it would take, then that's what it would have to be!

I heard Felix step on board. 'Make way, baguette, tartlets, fruit, milk, *charcuterie*…'

'Oh! You brought flowers! Aren't you a sweetie! Coffee coming right away, sir!'

I wiped my nose and gave him a big cheerful kiss.

'While I was on shore I thought I'd phone *le Professeur's* office for an appointment. We can see him tomorrow.'

My stomach sank. I hadn't expected to see *le Professeur* so soon. The letters had unsettled me and I knew I wouldn't sleep that night.

'Honey, I'm off to the *boulanger* and I'll phone Monique to wish her happy birthday while I'm ashore. She's home in the morning!'

I loved the short walk for our breakfast baguette. I liked to see the shop shutters go up, awnings roll down, waiters set out tables and chairs, and to breathe in the aroma of fresh coffee everywhere.

The fragrance of baking and fresh bread drifted well beyond the *boulangerie*. Inside, a cluster of women stood in a queue. We smiled and nodded. A sense of wellbeing filled the shop.

'*Bonjour, madame...comment ça va?*' The *boulanger* repeated again and again, to everyone.

I clutched my fresh stick, half wrapped in white tissue. I smelt it, broke off an end and munched the crunchy crust. How simple bliss can be! Then I remembered that in the afternoon we were seeing *le Professeur*. I pushed the thought aside and made for the telephone booth.

I checked my purse and pulled out all the coins I could use. Fortunately, I was phoning Lugano, not Australia. 'Hi Monique, this is Rina. Happy birthday. Don't weep. We all turn 60.'

'Aren't you marvellous to remember.'

'How could I forget my cousin's 60th birthday! Have a great day. Enjoy, enjoy.'

'How are things with you?'

'Well, we're seeing *le Professeur* this afternoon. I hope he says it's OK to move on. We're back from London, and the eye problem has nothing to do with the cancer, thank goodness.'

'You still sound apprehensive.'

'I guess I am, can't help it. Felix still can't read in the mornings although it's getting better. That's not a problem, I can do all the navigating, but he's not very steady on his legs. I guess I worry in case we get caught in a storm. But we plan just to sail along the coast. You know, from port to port. So we shouldn't get into trouble. We don't intend to cross to Corsica this year.'

'Can't you persuade Felix to give up and do something else?'

'Oh God, no! That would destroy him. You know, he's given up surgery, now he sees himself as a yachtie. I know there are other things he'd like to do, like study history, do a photography course, but that's not the same thing.'

'Yes, I guess you've got a point there.'

'I'll do anything for us to keep going, even if it entails risks. Anyway, I want to keep going just as much as Felix. Hey, Monique, I'm running out of coins. Have a wonderful birthday. And yes, there's life after 60. Give my love to André! Bye now!'

I put down the receiver and stepped out into the scorching heat.

'...So if you're feeling well, you can start on your way. But remember, don't climb the mast...' were *le Professeur's* parting words. In French, always in French. A tall, formal, elegant man with finely chiselled features, he extended his hand and smiled, '*Bonne chance*.' His handshake was firm and confident.

'Thank you for all your help,' Felix said when the two men shook hands.

As we crossed the window towards the door, I looked down onto a formal summer garden. 'Mediterranean gardens are so lovely,' I said.

'Yes, they are, so different with each season,' *le Professeur* replied. It was the first time he had loosened sufficiently to make an informal comment.

When we stepped outside, we didn't speak. Like guilty children, we were both aware that Felix hadn't told the Professor all he should have. Felix answered the questions but didn't mention his eyes. Neither of us wanted to risk advice we didn't want to hear. I was glad we'd parked the car a long way away — it was good to walk along the tree-lined street. We avoided talking about the consultation and concentrated on the colours and scents of the gardens, the twitter of birds in the trees.

'Let's go to the Place de la Comédie, and have coffee and *pâtisseries*. I'd like one of those almond and chocolate slices. And we can watch the passing parade and farewell Montpellier at the same time.'

Felix didn't hear. He wasn't listening. He looked concerned. 'When we get back, I'll change the oil and go over the engine. Nothing's been done for almost three months. Have to do that before we move off.'

So this, I realised, was to be his ultimate test — to see whether his hands were steady enough.

Felix removed the panels around the engine, then stretched out onto his side on the floor. 'I've got everything I need. You just shine the torch for me. Over here. Thanks, that's good. Pass me the pliers and the spanner and the WD-40. Thanks.'

'I think your most useful items to hold a boat together are shock cord and WD-40.'

'You're learning fast, kid.'

He was going through the list in the engine manual. I watched his hands nervously and followed them with the torch. They were steady.

'Now I'll just need to change the oil and top up the battery water and that'll be it.'

When he finally stood up and stretched, he beamed. I was right. This was the test he needed and he'd had no problems.

'The gas bottle we've been using must be just about empty, we'll need to change it. Could you write into the log book, "Changed oil, changed diesel filters. Battery water OK. Changed aft gas bottle."'

'I guess we're now ready to go. I'll settle the accounts at the *capitainerie*, and ask them to suggest where we can leave the car.'

Earlier that day we'd felt emotionally exhausted, but the relief had recharged our enthusiasm. We fell into each other's arms.

We walked up to the *capitainerie* to say goodbye. From the window, the outside was bathed in afternoon sunlight, the water a glitter of coloured lights. Along the pier *Galatea's* masts swayed from side to side as she slipped up and down with the swell. At her stern, fluttering in the breeze, was our Australian ensign and, on the port stay, the French courtesy flag.

'By the way, you can leave the car where it is until you're ready to pick it up,' Captain Alain said, 'and I've spoken to the *capitaineries* along the coast to make sure they help you when you radio that you are coming in. They will give you a hand. I don't think you should have any trouble.'

He said this nonchalantly, with a touch of embarrassment. He was a taciturn man, who rarely showed emotion. And yet, behind that façade, he was capable of such extraordinary thoughtfulness.

I shook hands with the captain and hugged Georges goodbye. What would we have done without their help?

'We'll aim to leave by midday,' Felix said.

'Do you think your eyes will be OK by then, or should we wait a little longer?'

'No, I should be fine by then.' In an afterthought, he added, 'Do you realise it's almost three months since our last sail?'

'Yes, I know,' and gave him a hug.

Felix turned on the engine and took the helm. I freed the ropes from the bollards, pushed out the bow, waved to the *capitainerie* and jumped on board. We motored past the port lights out to sea and hauled up all the sails. It was a cloudless day with a 10-knot nor'wester. Yet, in spite of the perfect conditions, we lacked our usual confidence and enthusiasm. The day was too momentous, and we were too apprehensive. We didn't go through our usual flippancies — the loud music, the singing along.

Close to the entrance to Les Saintes Mairies de la Mer, I radioed the *capitainerie*. A young man waited for us at the first pontoon. He waved us into a berth and caught our rope. 'We were expecting you, the *capitainerie* at Grande Motte let us know you were coming.'

'Yes, they are very kind, *merci beaucoup*.'

It was still hot when we tied up. Few people were outdoors, and unlike La Grande Motte, it was quiet. We sat in the cockpit for a while, relieved that this short sail had gone smoothly, then went ashore to visit the church.

The following morning Felix felt well, so we cast off early to avoid the midday heat and made for the group of islands — Iles de Ratonneau and Pomègues, 3 miles south-west of Marseilles. At various times, Phoenicians, Greeks and Romans had laid claim to them.

It was a clear morning with a good breeze, so we put up the sails and felt our old exuberance creep back. As we entered the Port du Frioul, our hearts skipped a beat. In a setting that looked more like a stage set than ancient ruins stood the erect pillars of a Roman temple, while on the horizon, a fully rigged, three-masted ship, its sails billowing, was gliding in an easterly direction.

We pulled into the marina and made fast. Two small sloops were tied to the pier, but there were no other signs of life. We felt an eerie sensation that we were intruders transported back in time. Apart from a marina, a few houses and a café at Port du Frioul, these islands were uninhabited.

At sunset, we climbed to the top of the hill for the spectacle that had brought so many impressionist painters here. As we sat on a rock high above Frioul, we watched the sun sink into the sea and felt Monet breathe over our shoulders.

We spent two days alone in this silent port. On one side of us was the sea, and on the other Marseilles unfolded and fanned out along the coast. In between, the Château d'If, a tiny island with stone fortifications, rose from the sea. Built four centuries earlier by François I for the defence of Marseilles, it was later used as a prison for political and religious captives. The Château d'If was now a tourist attraction for fans of *The Count of Monte Cristo*. Dumas chose a dramatic setting for his hero, one we now had to ourselves, away from the masses of twentieth century tourists who had turned this coastline into a fairground.

'I guess it's time to move on to Marseilles,' Felix said after two days.

The Romans called Marseilles the biggest whorehouse in the Mediterranean. Some maintain it has been the toughest and dirtiest place since time immemorial. Today many claim it is also the most crime-ridden town in France.

The most famous part of the port of Marseilles is its Vieux Port, where it all started, and around which the town expanded. While the rest of Marseilles has grown to keep up with the times, it has remained relatively unchanged, and retained its fabled romantic atmosphere for much of the twentieth century. But if a ghost were to visit his old stomping ground around the Vieux Port, he would now find pleasure yachts tied up to its pontoons, instead of the old clippers that had once plied the seas for trade. When I shut my eyes, I sensed the relief sailors must have felt to be home and safe here after weeks or months at sea. Even the drinking holes, we were told, had changed little.

We were lucky when we motored into the Vieux Port. Without asking for permission, we pulled into a berth just being vacated by a Dutch boat. A touch of chutzpah is not a bad thing sometimes. We asked for permission to tie up here *after* we were safely ensconced. As we were pulling into the marina, we noticed a young man observing us with interest. When we returned from the office he seemed anxious to talk.

'I notice you have an Australian flag. Was your boat built in Australia?'

'Yes,' Felix replied.

'I have never seen a boat built in Australia. Would you mind if I come on board and have a look?' We were taken aback but were reluctant to say no. He looked respectable enough — in his 20s, dark hair, clean-shaven, neat, in a pair of beige slacks, brown boat shoes and a striped T-shirt. It hadn't occurred to us that he might be a druggie, a criminal or that he might have had an ulterior motive for looking over the boat. Yet there was something about him that made us uncomfortable. Perhaps it was the unusual French he spoke. But then along the coast there were so many newcomers from Africa whose accents varied, depending on where they came from.

Once on board, however, he chatted about Marseilles but gave nothing away about himself. Then he asked whether he could have a drink. 'So how long do you expect to stay in Marseilles?' He settled himself on the settee and we wondered how long he was likely to stay. We were anxious to go ashore.

'Oh, just a couple of days. We intend to move along the coast for another three weeks. Then we plan to leave the boat somewhere near here for the winter. Do you know a marina where we could do that?'

As soon as I'd said this, I realised I'd made a mistake, and appreciated the fact that Felix didn't kick me under the table.

'Oh yes, no problem, I'll talk to a friend I have and I'll come back this evening and let you know.' It was all very promising. He had drunk the best part of a bottle but appeared unaffected.

'Meet me at that bar over there,' he pointed to a bar on the Quay du Port, 'at 9 o'clock this evening and I'll be able to give you all the information.'

After he'd left we were still not at ease, but strangely pleased to have met someone who could help us find a wintering place for *Galatea*. We walked to the end of the marina to inspect the offerings in the fish market at the Quay des Belges, a mistake on a hot day. To flee the smell, we quickly trotted off towards the bars, cafés and pizzerias near the Quay de Rive Neuve.

We settled into cane chairs under the blue awning of a small café overlooking the water. Culinary odours drifted onto the footpath, and French *chansons* filled the airwaves. A waiter floated effortlessly from table to table, and with a professional sweep of his arm, presented us with the menu. We ordered eggplant fritters and half a carafe of white house wine. At a table next to us sat a middle-aged man with a navy beret, smoking a pipe, a glass of wine in one hand and a newspaper in the other.

At another table, a German couple with a dachshund were eating pasta and drinking red wine. The eggplant fritters were still sizzling when the waiter put our plates down.

'Umm, delicious. Crisp on the outside, soft on the inside.'

We sipped the wine and continued to sit and gaze over the marina, taking deep breaths of sea air spiced with a touch of fish odour, and reflecting on our good fortune.

'Let's move on and have coffee where the action is,' Felix suggested.

The Canebière is Marseilles's main fashionable avenue, where people lounge in outdoor cafés and restaurants, and elegant women promenade between shops. We went in search of *pâtisseries* and espressos.

We returned to *Galatea* at 6.30 to shower before our appointment with the young man whose name we had carelessly forgotten to ask.

By now the Vieux Port and the area surrounding it were a blaze of bright lights. Preened people stepped off boats for the night's entertainment. I was apprehensive, but Felix didn't let on whether he was.

As we neared the bar, the music was deafening. Young men with black hair and sharp eyes filled the bar and the outdoor tables. I felt them stare in a puzzled way as we made for an empty table in a corner. It was the seediest bar on that strip. Felix and I looked at each other.

'What will you drink?' a grim waiter asked in a gruff tone.

'Mineral water,' I said, too frightened to ask for any-thing else.

'A Carlsberg beer,' Felix said.

The men kept turning to look at us. The language they spoke was unlike the French we were used to.

'I want to get away,' I whispered.

'We can't, the bloke should be here any minute. He said 9 o'clock. We said we'd be here.'

'I don't care what he's arranged, we shouldn't have anything to do with him.'

'Sure, we won't have anything to do with him, but it may be unwise for us not to wait and at least pretend that we're going to leave *Galatea* with his friend.'

We continued to whisper.

'Do you want anything to eat?' the waiter snapped.

'Do you have pizza?'

'Yes,' was the sharp reply. He walked away before we'd told him what kind of a pizza we wanted.

In spite of the cool breeze, I was in a bath of sweat. While we waited, a gaggle of women in miniskirts, stiletto patent boots and thick masks of paint roared into the bar and distributed themselves among the tables. Some sat on the men's laps, others made for high stools at the bar. The men stopped staring at us and now focused on the girls. It was after 10.

Our pizzas arrived. 'What if they're laced?' I wasn't hungry.

'I doubt it,' Felix looked starved.

'How long are we going to wait?'

'We'll just eat the pizzas and then leave.'

By the time we finished it was 10.30 and the young man still hadn't come. We paid. The waiter looked relieved when he saw us walk out the door.

We walked in silence back to the marina. The restaurants were busy, and there was frenetic activity all around. Lights blazed along the quay, yachts rocked, booms swayed, rigging chimed, but few people were around. Almost everyone was ashore.

We climbed on board.

'Thank God we can go to bed. Let's leave at the crack of dawn.'

'Don't turn,' Felix whispered, 'but I think the guy is at the end of this pier with his back to us.' He put the key into the lock of the washboard.

'Someone's been tampering with the lock. Look at the scratches, the lock's bent! I can't get the key in. I'll need a screwdriver and pliers.'

My stomach sank. 'Maybe we forgot to lock the workshop from the inside.'

We were in luck. We raised the cockpit seat. Felix climbed in and came out with a screwdriver and a pair of pliers, and opened the lock.

'I can't believe we were such idiots. We've just fallen for the oldest con in the book!' Felix said with a smile.

I insisted we lock ourselves in.

Early the next morning we went to the marina office to pay.

'You want to go to Cassis with your boat? But *c'est impossible* to go in…too many people…' the official at the Vieux Port *capitainerie* insisted.

'Maybe we'll be lucky.' Felix resisted telling him that our greatest concern was to get out of Marseilles as fast as we could.

◎◎◎◎

It was already afternoon when we approached the lighthouse at Cassis, not a good time to find a spot on the marina. Nevertheless, I radioed the *capitainerie*. Some minutes later I called out to Felix, 'Yes, they know about us. They'll send someone to the entrance to give us a hand. They said it's really crowded but they'll squeeze us in somewhere. God bless Captain Alain.'

At the entrance a young man gesticulated instructions. We had furled the sails, turned on the engine, and were moving slowly in the direction of the quay where hulls were glued cheek to cheek.

'You're jolly lucky to come in before the Mistral hits,' an English voice from the boat alongside greeted us.

It was a tight fit on the marina, the fenders between the boats groaned. We were squeezed between a Scandinavian and a chatty Englishman. When we told him how concerned we were about finding a place to winter *Galatea*, he said, 'You should've arranged a wintering spot at least three months ago. If I were you, I'd try and find a spot on the hard instead of leaving her in the water on a marina. Around Marseilles pilfering and robbing is a standard occupation. Much safer to be on the dry in a fenced and guarded compound. If you like, I'll give you the phone number of the Port Sec at Martigues where I'm leaving my boat.'

We were grateful for the advice, phoned the following morning and secured a wintering spot from the first week in October.

Towards evening, we walked past the commotion of the quay and the restaurants into a quiet area, where an old world atmosphere pervaded a tiny park. With geometric flowerbeds of red geraniums, white chrysanthemums, yellow marigolds and daisies, the scene was a Renoir vignette. An aged couple bent over a stone table were playing cards, a grey-haired woman sat on a bench embroidering a tablecloth, children clutching twigs chased each other on gravel paths. This was not the tourists' Cassis. That centred on the quay, and in the restaurants.

Monet, Matisse, Dufy, Vlaminck and Derain had all fallen in love with Cassis, a village nestling at the end of a bay where escarpments sweep down to the sea. When the painters had come here, it was a fishing community.

That evening the Mistral hit with a vengeance. At the entrance to the port the sea was angry, and the wind whistled, but our corner was relatively still. It was good to get into our bunks. We took out our eiderdowns, and the next morning breakfasted on porridge with brown sugar for the first time. We had come to France in early spring, spent the summer there, and now we were well into autumn.

'If the Mistral is going to blow for a few days, we could pick up the car and visit wineries, go to Aix-en-Provence and other places.' When he wasn't exhausted, Felix needed to keep moving. Perhaps this was a way of proving to himself that he still had the energy, that he was almost back to normal.

By the time we had caught two buses and one train, it had taken us over eight hours to bring our car from La Grande Motte to Cassis.

On the following day, armed with a *Michelin Green Guide*, a *Michelin Red Guide*, Hugh Johnson's *Wine Atlas of France,* and maps of Provence and the Côte d'Azur, we set off well after midday, the time of day when Felix, like Proust, felt he could face the world. I wore a big straw hat, not only to cover my hair but also to cut down the number of migraines that plagued me. When I wore my large red number, people at the marina christened me '*la dame au chapeau rouge*'.

Our first excursion was along the coastal road between Cassis and Ciotat — a steep, winding road overlooking the water and villages below. The sea and sky were a moving kaleidoscope in shades of blues, greens, greys and whites. The countryside was autumnal. Trees were heavy with fruit and leaves were turning gold. The vintage was in full swing. We drove along narrow byways overgrown with branches, past hidden road signs (frequently pointing in the wrong direction) to Moulin des Costes near La Cadière d'Azur. Felix wanted to talk about

French wines, but the vignerons wanted to discuss Australian ones. They looked astonished when we told them that we had no home address, and that the wines we bought would be stored in the bilge of our boat. After a short silence, they refilled our glasses and said, '*C'est vraiment formidable*, we are jealous!'

'I never knew there were so many people in the world who'd like to live on a boat but don't,' I said to Felix as we lugged two boxes into the boot. We drove on to Domaine de Pibarnon, bought another dozen reds and then climbed to Le Castellet, a quaint village nestled on a peak with a panoramic vista over the plain below.

'Ah, how Cezanne loved this place!' The restaurateur told us.

It was still blowing a gale when we set off to Aix-en-Provence and parked off the boulevard in the centre of town. Cours Mirabeau is a wide boulevard, lined with cafés and rows of massive plane trees planted three centuries ago.

'There's a café in the shade, it looks like a university campus eatery, let's go there,' I said. It was packed, but a young man invited us to sit with him and his friend. 'The advantage of looking old,' I muttered to Felix.

It didn't take long to start a conversation. They spoke fluent English, German and French. The two were a contrast in looks and manner. Reinhardt, the younger of the two, was fair-haired, cheerful, slight and gregarious. Werner was tall, dark, heavy and formal. He pulled out a chair for me and we shook hands.

Reinhardt was happy to tell us what they were doing in Aix-en-Provence. 'We're both law students from Munich, studying European and international law here. That's going to be very important in the future. We're studying here because it'll improve our French and also we'll learn legalese French. It won't be easy to combine all the various national systems into a European one.

That's why we're encouraged to study in other countries, not just in Germany. We've been here a year and we'll stay another year. Provence is a great place. A bit like a holiday really.'

Werner was more anxious to tell us what we should see in Aix-en-Provence: '…you must see Cezanne's Atelier, it's open till 6…and of course you must walk through Old Aix. It's a place with boulevards, squares, museums, a sprawling university housed in old buildings, Gothic and Renaissance architecture, cafés, good food and a long history.'

Cezanne's Studio, a house and garden at the top of a steep hill, was just as it had been when he died in 1906. We were the only visitors that day. To see the blue vase, the water jug, the plaster cupid — all items we'd seen in his paintings — was a moving experience. I touched the easel and imagined I smelt his paint.

After the Mistral had blown itself out, we continued on to St Tropez for several days. In early October we bid *Galatea* a sad farewell on the dry at Martigues and drove through a golden French autumn to London. We were looking forward to seeing our two granddaughters, who were going to spend their school holidays with us.

'Well, that's the end of our first summer!'

'Quite a summer,' Felix replied.

'Yes, and we'll have a great winter in London. Renting a flat near Swiss Cottage tube station will be handy. Think of all the concerts and theatres and galleries…and taking the girls out, I can't wait.'

'We'll also have to find out what 9- and 12-year-old girls enjoy doing.'

◎ ◎ ◎ ◎

chapter four

⊚ ⊚ ⊚ ⊚

Hi Kids!

It's April, and we're in France on our way south at the start of our second summer. You should see us! Our car is packed to the roof. New mattresses for the saloon, more nautical technology, books and tapes, and we're making our way slowly to *Galatea*.

We're well, the spring countryside is as magnificent as these enclosed photos but you're lucky the smell doesn't come with them. We keep the car windows closed. Dad's convinced we've run over a cow or two and that's why we can't get away from it.

But we are definitely eating and drinking our way south. Dinner yesterday: asparagus soufflé, *quenelles de brochet* (pike), ham with mushroom cream sauce, raspberry soufflé. But we pay for this bliss with my nightly rashes. Dad's eyes have improved, but he can't use a pen so he'll write when he gets to the computer.

We loved John Ardagh's *Writers' France*. It's a wonderful guide to the homes and places where famous writers lived or spent time. It was especially thrilling to visit the house where Marcel Proust had that famous incident of the madeleine soaked in tea (now that we've both finished his three tomes). Of course as soon as we shut the front gate, we rushed to the nearest café to have madeleines, but can you believe, they gave us coffee instead of tea!

We drove on through the Beuce, Émile Zola's territory, and finally to the Château de Saché where Balzac spent most of his time writing in bed. It's a great way to amble through the French countryside in spring.

We miss getting letters from you, but we'll phone when we get to Martigues and *Galatea*. Hope you're all well.

Lots of love and hugs from us both

It was good to arrive in Martigues, put *Galatea* into the water and sleep in a familiar environment. After a week spent getting her shipshape, we moved from port to port along the coast to Villefranche and St Jean Cap Ferrat. We picked up the car from Martigues, and while we waited for David to pass through on his way to a conference, we familiarised ourselves with the coast and hinterland of this part of France.

We drove several times to the Fondation Maeght, a wonderful gallery on the way to our favourite, St Paul de Vence, where Chagall spent the last 30 years of his life. We visited the Chagall Museum, the Picasso Museum in Antibes, Matisse's Chapel in Vence…We celebrated our 40th wedding anniversary with David in Juan-les-Pins, where we dined on a nine-course degustation menu and drank innumerable toasts.

'Let's have a family celebration here for our 50th wedding anniversary,' I said, and crossed my fingers. At midnight we needed a taxi to get back to *Galatea*.

On the French Riviera we met an Englishman who had lived there for many years. He was a tall, lanky man in his 60s with a handlebar moustache, thinning, mottled grey hair, a smart upright gait and clipped upper crust accent. In an earlier era he would have felt at home in India, spent his leisure time at the officers' club, and eventually retired to Tunbridge Wells. Indeed, he reminded us of the quintessential British expat portrayed in books about India. But of course, he was much too young to have been one. Still, he invariably assumed an air of superiority whenever he alluded to non-Brits.

We first met Alistair on the marina in Beaulieu, where he spent much of his time trolling for novices, preferably those planning to cross to Calvi for the first time, with whom he could share his extensive knowledge of Corsica, where he had a house. He took pleasure in visiting us almost daily during the weeks we spent on marinas in, or close to, Beaulieu. If we wanted to have a day to ourselves we moved out of the marina and anchored in one of the bays, such as Villefranche, or more often, drove off inland, and on occasion, to Italy for the day. We found it strange that, in all the time he'd lived in the South of France, he had never ventured further than Corsica.

Alistair admitted on a number of occasions that he didn't like France or the French, yet never offered a reason why he lived there, other than admitting that '…the weather is so damn good'. He didn't like Corsicans either (although he loved Corsica), and he never missed an occasion to warn us about their 'perfidious habits'.

'Buy a Corsican flag and fly it!' he advised us. We did — a 'Tête de Maure, a Moor's Head' flag, originally used by the Aragonese during the Crusades and later adopted by Corsican patriots. Alistair had stayed in all the 'anses' (bays and inlets), on the west coast of Corsica, which, he assured us, was far more picturesque than the east coast. He also knew a great deal about the British who lived on the French Riviera, and advised them on buying property in the South of France.

'There's an entire colony of British who are permanent residents here, and we mingle primarily among ourselves...' We never met Alistair's wife, although he professed to have one. She played a lot of bridge, he said.

It was the longest day of the year, with a full silver moon, the day we cast off from the marina of Beaulieu. On Alistair's advice we left at 2 in the afternoon to ensure sighting Punta Revellata lighthouse at dawn. This was the first time we were leaving a coastline and crossing a stretch of water. Although I knew that in a storm it was safer to be out at sea than close to land, I felt more secure hugging a coast.

Our flags hung limp and the engine purred as we waved Alistair goodbye. The sun was burning deep orange and yellow, and along the coast there was frenetic activity. By sunset, however, we felt an evening breeze and switched off the engine.

'What's for dinner? I'm starved, we must open an appropriate wine for the occasion.'

'A cheese soufflé and a baguette. Something light for the crossing,' I said. 'And raspberries with nougat gelato to follow.'

'Perfect.'

The sky was cloudless, a full moon had slipped above the horizon, but the occasion was too emotional for our bravura singalong. By 10 o'clock it was dark, the moon was high, stars glittered, and we drifted on in silence. We stayed in the cockpit all night; neither of us contemplated going to bed.

'We should see the Revellata light soon.'

I drifted off to sleep in the cockpit and woke with a start when Felix announced, 'There's the light! Earlier than I thought, it's just after 3.'

'And all we did was point the autohelm to 138 degrees and we're almost in Corsica!'

Just then two yachts crossed our path on their way north, and in the distance a cruise ship, lit up like a carnival ball, was making its way towards the Italian coast.

Gradually, the mist enveloping the Corsican coast lifted, and an outline of the Calvi citadel appeared. Built by the Genoese in the thirteenth century, it sits perched on a tall escarpment at the entrance to Calvi harbour. We entered the port at 5.30. Not a soul was in sight. At about 7, the place came to life. Set among palms, the bars and cafés opened, and people started to step ashore from boats.

The port was noisy and busy, its dominant feature the view of the citadel above. In the evenings, the restaurants and bars were packed when uniformed Foreign Legion conscripts came down from the citadel for a night's entertainment with the local girls.

The atmosphere in Calvi — its sounds and smells, the whitewashed houses with their bright-coloured doors and flowerpots — is more Italian than French. The ancient town, which has a 600-year history, is perched up on the citadel. It was eerily still and silent when we climbed the steep walk to see it. The houses that had once been whitewashed looked forlorn and uninhabited, yet that couldn't be. The Foreign Legion had barracks there, but we didn't see any of the conscripts. We only saw an old woman on a stool in front of an open door, her head tilted back, sunning herself, and a cat curled at her feet. The smell of cooking drifted into the air.

We hired a car and drove inland. Much of the landscape is harsh and rugged, and according to guide books, not lacking in *banditi*: '...never stare or get involved in anything that seems strange or unusual.' On the Route de Bavella — famous for its spectacular needle peaks, known as *Aiguilles de Bavella* — pine and chestnut trees, wild pigs and boars abound. Large expanses are covered with aromatic herbs and shrubs (*maquis*), and when the wind blows off the land, exotic scents sweep as far as 20 miles out to sea.

The island has been described as 'a scented granite mountain surrounded by anchorages'. The west coast, from Calvi to Ajaccio, is mountainous, with deep, steep-sided bays and inlets. Most have small beaches and crystal water with shimmering kaleidoscope colours, perfect for anchoring and peaceful interludes. Many resemble alpine lakes surrounded by mountains. The names are mostly Italian — Girolata, Propriano, Campo Moro, Tizzano, Roccapina. Ruins of towers, citadels and small settlements sprinkle the coastline. Some look like villages, but are in fact mausoleums that look like housing estates. One had a golden cupola, a small version of St Peter's Basilica. It was built over 100 years ago by a Corsican who had migrated to South America. His descendants are still brought here for burial. These edifices — like lighthouses, forts and other remarkable features in the landscape — are marked on naval charts.

Although the inlets were filled with yachts in the summer months, they were quiet. Everyone, it seemed to us, was addicted to 'The Ritual of Bronzage'. People lay motionless on the beach or on the back of boats equipped with thick mattresses. The procedure was to baste and rotate every twenty minutes. Only a cigarette, lunch or a call of nature induced anyone to suspend 'thinking Bronzage'. And so the days passed. After dark, lights from portholes glittered on rippled water, yachts rocked on shafts of moonlight, and the bay was silent.

The approaches to Bonifacio, on the southern tip of Corsica, resemble an exotic geological formation a billion years old, indented with steep escarpments, caves and grottos. We couldn't work out where to turn in. Finally, we followed an island ferry, on the assumption that its captain had made it to the entrance before. We had never seen anything like Bonifacio harbour.

The old town is inside the fortress at the top of a daunting escarpment, which has views over the harbour below, and across the Straits of Bonifacio to Sardinia, a few miles away. 'An ideal harbour for pirates and bandits,' Felix said.

But most of the action was at sea level when we were there. The marina was at the end of the long, deep, fjord-like bay, with many indents where yachts tied up against rock faces.

We were ingenues when we arrived in Corsica, and had to acquire special Mediterranean skills. Soon after leaving Calvi, a breeze filled our sails and we drifted on in silence. There was no vessel in sight, and we were both reading. Now and again we looked up at the beauty of the sea and coastline, and felt as if we were alone in the world. After a long spell of such bliss, I went down to prepare lunch. Suddenly, the deafening silence was shattered by a 'SHWUSSH' and a loud 'SHIT!!!'

I popped my head out just as a sailing vessel slipped past our stern, and a slim naked bottom stared me in the face. The shock sent my pulse racing. This palest of bottoms turned to reveal a full frontal view of a bearded young man, with long hair, pained dark eyes and outstretched arms.

'Jesus Christ!' I cried out.

'That wasn't Jesus Christ. It's a metal boat, and had it been sailing 5 degrees further east it would have sliced through us!' Felix was in a state of shock.

'I've never seen such a shocked naked man with arms outstretched. I thought it was a Visitation!'

Felix didn't think this was funny. The near sinking horrified him.

Neither the young man nor we had been keeping watch. His boom hit our stays, and his sail swept our sail, on an open, empty sea. It was a salutary, close shave.

'OK. From now on,' Felix decreed, 'only one of us reads. The other stays on watch!'

Most of our Mediterranean learning experiences related to methods of tying or untying at odd quays or rock walls. Sometimes we had to go in bow first, at other times stern first. Our most exciting attempt prompted a young Frenchman to risk his life. He dived off his boat, caught our line, which was much too short for our purpose, lengthened it with a rope he supplied, and tied it to a steep rock face in Bonifacio.

Later that day, when a ferocious wind hit and he had to move to the other side, he wouldn't let us untie his rope and return it to him. '*Pas de problème*, no problem,' he assured us. '*Demain*, give it back tomorrow.'

Some days later, when it looked as if we were going to be blown onto a different constellation of rocks, another Frenchman rescued us by jumping into his dinghy and taking our anchor out.

'There must be advantages in looking old, frail and foreign. But we need to make a list of our problems,' I concluded. 'OK. Our problems are due to:

1 Not having the anchor ready.
2 Not having the chain locker open.
3 Not having the dinghy prepared and tied to the bow.
4 Not having adequate ropes ready.
5 Not having the anchor winch turned on.

'Lists, Puss, there's nothing like making lists for every contingency and sticking them on the appropriate wall close to the gangway.'

By the time we reached the first island between Corsica and Sardinia, our style had definite panache. But we still needed to learn how to deal with 'spaghetti anchor lines'.

In many ports in Italy, unlike France, it was customary to tie up to the public quay. The method was to drop the anchor a long way out, then back the boat up to the quay, squeeze in between two boats, and tie up. We managed that without anyone needing to risk their lives for us.

By evening other boats had done the same, but when there was no room on the quay, boats tied up to the boat in front of them. Sometimes half a dozen were tied one behind the other, and anchor lines and chains criss-crossed. At first we were naïve enough to tie up to the quay whenever possible, but the traffic of people stepping back and forth across *Galatea's* deck at all hours of the night was brisk, and each time they stepped on board, we were woken with: '*Permesso*, sorry, *pardon*, *entschuldigung...*'

If we planned to leave early in the morning, we had to allow up to two hours to untangle the anchor lines. Watching other people untangle these in a mixture of languages and temperaments certainly did afford a morning's entertainment. On the deck of every boat onlookers tried to assist: '...*si, si, un poco a destra*, a little to the right, *poco piu*, a little more, *nein, nein...mais non, un petit peu à droite*, a little bit to the right...'

The first time we found ourselves on an Italian quay and had not yet mastered the exercise, Felix watched and studied the technique. Soon he'd convinced himself that 'we're not the only idiots'. And when we pulled out of the marina at La Maddalena, our manoeuvres were so expert we couldn't resist beaming from ear to ear.

'Porto Cervo in Sardinia is a *must!'* we were told. 'It's the most expensive marina in Christendom, the Aga Khan's playground. Guaranteed by arrangement, no kidnapping during summer months. But for goodness sake, don't tie up at the marina. It'll cost you an arm and a leg. You can put down an anchor in the bay and go ashore in the dinghy.'

Armed with this piece of information, we made for Sardinia. First to Porto Liscia, then Porto Pollo, a crystal bay where we went slightly aground and were pulled off by another yacht, and then on to Porto Cervo where we anchored in the roadstead, a large bay, among bigger and more glamorous boats.

Porto Cervo was the first Italian port where we could request the mandatory boat documentation, the *constituzio,* to sail in Italian waters. While Felix set off to the *capitaineria di porto,* I bought myself a *Herald Tribune* and the most expensive cappuccino I'd ever had and waited. Felix returned after an hour.

'The officer-in-charge didn't stop talking about Australia. Of course he has relatives there. In Melbourne and in Perth. As for the *constituzio*, he said nothing will happen to us if we don't have one. He said it was really hot today. Too hot to bother. He suggested we should get one in Elba. And now I need a cappuccino.'

'Sure, but don't ask how much they charge.'

The next day we moved on and anchored in a nearby quiet bay. The weather was magnificent and the water still, when a young man in a dinghy, obviously despatched from the marina, came alongside *Galatea* in the late afternoon to tell us there was a severe storm forecast for the night. 'You should come into the marina. It will be safer for you…' We found this very thoughtful. But it was a clear, still evening and when we turned on the radio for a forecast, there was no mention of storms. So we decided to chance it and stayed.

It was a starlit, idyllic night. Apart from the occasional grumble of the anchor chain, there was no movement at all. Later, we realised the 'storm warning' was a regular ploy used to fill marinas. We'd mastered tying up against rock faces, but we still had a lot to learn.

A steady 20-knot wind, gusting 30, zoomed us from Sardinia north to Porto-Vecchio in Corsica. The air was a veil of sapphire. Needles of spray pricked our faces as *Galatea* cut the waves and raced the wind towards the Gulf, where shades of blue tinted each layer of the mountain range.

'It's like a Chinese landscape painting.'

It was a long, steep walk to Porto-Vecchio village at the top of the escarpment. In the central village square, waiters with trays held high flitted between tables under pergolas smothered in creepers. The scent of jasmine and sea filled the air. Old men played chess and cards, visitors read papers and everyone drank wine or coffee.

'Apart from tourists and the marina, I bet nothing's changed here for centuries.'

'There's something attractive about little change.'

We bought a paper, sipped wine and stretched our legs.

'It was a fabulous sail today, Puss. But it's even better to sit still now.'

Felix smiled. 'Enjoy stretching your legs. Tomorrow we should move to St Cyprien at the northern end of the Gulf, and leave from there for Elba after midnight.'

On our last night in Corsica, Felix spent a long time taking sights of the numerous rocks around us, then bent over the navigation table and, with parallel rule, dividers and 2B pencil in hand, plotted our course out of St Cyprien.

'It's going to be pitch black, no moon, and we'll have to go out of here entirely on radar. That way we'll only have four hours with no visibility. It'll dawn at about 5,' Felix reassured me.

We weighed anchor shortly after 1 am. Although Felix was confident and in complete control as we moved between boulders that neither of us could see, I found the exercise nerve-racking. It was black, not even a shore light in view. I sat in the cockpit, and kept my eyes on the tiny red radar light. *Galatea* was creaking and groaning, as aware of the rocks as I was.

As soon as we had cleared the rocks I relaxed, and set the autohelm on a 40-degree course for Elba.

'Do we now have a late supper or early breakfast?'

'Whichever is bigger,' Felix replied.

'Welsh rarebit?'

'Great.'

Coffee was already in the thermos. We ate in the cockpit, with our eyes glued to the radar screen. Three small ships moved across the screen in different directions.

'I wish it'd start to dawn.'

'It will, sooner than you think.' Felix put his arm around me.

To see the dawn creep and sweep away the night's blackness is as heady as sailing under a brilliant moon. The first thin stripe of colour lined the eastern sky as the island of Monte Cristo appeared on radar. Soon after, an arc of brilliant yellow peeped over the horizon, and the sky changed slowly from dark grey to mandarin and pink. Then, the grey outlines of Monte Cristo and its neighbouring island of Pianosa came into view, both set against a pink sky.

We sailed on. The sea had now changed from black to dark blue, the morning breeze had stiffened, and our wake trailed and spun like a cord. The sun was high when Elba appeared under a cloudless sky. We made for Porto Azzurro.

We furled the sails at the entrance to the harbour, turned on the engine and looked at the crowded quay. 'Let's tie up behind that Austrian boat. There are only two in front of her.'

'It's 4.30, just over fifteen hours. It was a good crossing. No drama.'

We dropped anchor and motored slowly up to the yacht flying an Austrian flag. The couple on board stood on their aft deck and helped us tie up.

'Did you come from Corsica?'

'Yes, we've spent the last two weeks in Corsica and Sardinia.'

'What's the food like in Corsica?'

'Jams are great,' I said, 'but sometimes I think Corsican food and wine were the reasons Napoleon fled to France.'

I wasn't surprised they asked about the food. They looked like hearty eaters.

'Where have you come from?' Felix asked.

'Tuscany. It's beautiful but very crowded. We hope to find some quiet spots on the islands. Here in Porto Azzurro it's very noisy. Portoferraio and anywhere on the other side of Elba is much better. We're on our way to Greece for a few months. Maybe also Turkey…Come over and have a drink with us!'

I was beat, but Felix wanted to talk to them about Tuscany, so we joined them.

Among yachties, the conversation invariably centred on where one had been, advice on where to go, where not to go, and an exchange of hair-raising stories. At this stage of our travels, we were mainly the recipients of advice. So we chatted for a while until they noticed that I was ready to drop. 'We'll let you rest. Enjoy Elba.'

Portoferraio is a great spot as long as you don't tie up at the noisy quay. We anchored in the roadstead instead, and from there had a view of the whole long saddle of the town. On our own, in the middle of the bay, we swung on our anchor chain, and pointed into the wind. The breeze swept through the front hatch, and seagulls perched on the crosstrees on the lookout for crumbs.

Each day we motored to the quay by dinghy, had coffee in the main square, read the *Herald Tribune* and watched the passing parade. Sometimes, we motored in for a stroll and meal in the evening. T-shirts were our new fascination. No matter what the nationality of the wearer, the inscriptions were always in English. 'I love NY', 'I love LA', 'I love San Fran' but never 'I love Rome' or 'J'aime Paris'.

When enough time had elapsed for our mail to be couriered to Elba, we set off on our daily mission to the post office. But each day the people at the counter stared at us as if we'd come from a planet where mail was delivered regularly, even at the height of summer.

'It was sent by courier!' We argued.

'But in summer the couriers are on holiday!' they said.

'It's useless,' I said to Felix as we stepped into the dinghy to motor home.

Napoleon was mad, we decided. He lived up on the hill overlooking the bay, in the Palazzina dei Mulini, for just ten months from May 1814, when he reigned over this small kingdom. Apart from this 'town palace', where he lived with his mother and sister, he had a summerhouse.

'Napoleon was not only mad, but greedy, and bored as well. After all, for a loser he didn't do too badly. A beautiful island, lots of beaches, two houses…' I said.

'Ah! Ambitious and in need of *Lebensraum*, space.'

Elba is a 'safe-feeling' kind of place with a gentle landscape, different from the wild rugged beauty of Corsica and Sardinia. Italians who live in Tuscany use Elba as we'd used Broken Bay, north of Sydney. It's easy to find shelter for boats, there are numerous beaches, and it's possible to get away from crowds and swim in crystal water.

'Maybe we could find a wintering place for *Galatea* here?'

We were amazed when the first boatyard we investigated was owned by an Australian. 'Yes, I guess you are surprised,' he said. 'When I finished school in Melbourne, I decided to come and live in Italy where my parents had come from. I love living in Elba…' But Elba was packed and he couldn't help us.

'It's mid-August and time to move on to the mainland…' Felix said as we made our way yet again to the post office.

'Yes, on to Tuscany!'

◎◎◎◎

All the private marinas in Viareggio were packed. We had no alternative but to tie up in the ugly industrial marina, with a large Saudi yacht undergoing massive renovations on one side of us and a clapped out yacht with a charming poodle on the other. But we didn't mind — it was free, it was easy to get the refrigerator gassed and minor repairs done, and in any case, we were ready to move on and start our sentimental journey north along the Italian Riviera.

The eastern half of the Italian Riviera, the *Riviera di Levante* — with its promontories, inlets, bays and villages — has attracted painters, writers and poets for centuries. Lerici, at the foot of a steep incline that slopes down to a horseshoe bay in the Gulf of La Spezia, is now both a fishing village and a tourist resort. Dante was an early visitor to Lerici. Many English exiles who had chosen to live in Italy spent time here. For early nineteenth century romantics, Italy was 'the paradise of exiles', where they hoped to experiment with new forms of life and new rules. Many writers and poets, like Byron and Shelley, had chosen to lead 'gypsy lives', for which Felix and I had a newly acquired understanding.

In 1822 Shelley lived here in the hope of improving his health, but alas, drowned when his boat sank in bad weather. His many literary friends felt the need to give him a dramatic send-off. So, in the presence of Byron, Leigh Hunt, Trelawny, local militia and fishermen, Shelley was cremated. A copy of Keats's poems was thrown onto the pyre. Byron, in an emotional state, swam 3 miles out to his yacht, the *Bolivar*, and back. After the cremation, Trelawny raked out Shelley's heart and gave it Byron, who passed it on to Leigh Hunt, who in turn gave it to Shelley's wife Mary. Trelawny knew that Byron would have liked Shelley's skull, but remembering that Byron had once used a skull as a drinking vessel, decided not to give it to him.

The stretch of coastline from Viareggio north to the Gulf of La Spezia, Lerici and Portovenere had been a stomping ground for these English Romantics. But the closest we came to feeling the Romantics' presence was a café called the Café Byron, and also a plaque in Portovenere that commemorates Byron in grandiloquent language: '…the immortal poet who as a daring swimmer defied the waves of the sea from Portovenere to Lerici'. I imagine this impressed the villagers more than the English exiles' experiments in new forms of living. We continued north, past the Cinque Terre — the five fishing villages set in narrow, shallow inlets — towards our destination, Portofino.

For us, Portofino will always stir memories of that summer's day in 1953 when we had vowed that some day we'd have our own boat and sail the Mediterranean.

Some months beforehand, we'd arrived in London from Australia in a cargo ship. Felix had signed up as ship's surgeon in exchange for a free passage. Our official reason for coming to England was to further Felix's surgical training, to get his FRCS (Fellowship of the Royal College of Surgeons), but our real agenda was to see the world. We were young, adventurous and impecunious. At the end of Felix's first hospital stint as a surgical resident, we crossed the English Channel and made for the South of France and Italy.

Instead of taking the road out of Santa Margherita to Rapallo, we erred onto a narrow winding road that led us past views over a jagged coastline and a glittering sea. By the time we realised that we'd taken a wrong turn, the scenery and the scents led us to a village nestled at the end of a horseshoe bay.

Tall, terraced houses in shades of ochre, pink, yellow and terracotta lined the inlet. At the entrance was a cobbled piazza clogged with stalls selling food, clothing, tablecloths, pots and pans. The place buzzed with shrieks of laughter, and smelt of fish, cheeses, fruit and vegetables. The women, many dressed in long skirts, were coarse-skinned; the men, in baggy trousers and fishermen's hats, had weathered faces.

'Do you think we're the only strangers here?' I whispered to Felix.

'Can't see anyone looking foreign.'

As we wandered among the stalls, people looked at us with curiosity. We bought peaches, then moved on to the quay. Two luxury yachts were tied up there; one belonged to the Duke and Duchess of Windsor, we heard someone say. But apart from these, only rowing boats and sailing dinghies bobbed up and down along the quayside. An old fisherman, his hands crippled with arthritis, was gathering his nets.

'*Inglesi?*' He smiled.

'No, *Australiani*.'

'*Australiani?*' he said, his voice full of amazement. '*Mio zio* in Australia...had an uncle...went there before the first war... Australia *è lontano*, a long way...*Tempi erano difficili*...times were hard.'

We offered to help him fold his sail. He was grateful. As we helped, we talked in my hesitant Italian. I told him about the dinghy we sailed in Sydney Harbour.

The piazza had almost emptied when he said, 'Would you like to take out my boat? I've finished fishing today. You can tie it up when you come back, and I'll come down in the evening.' Felix and I looked at each other and didn't know how to respond. Then after a short silence, Felix looked at the man and said, '*Grazie, tanto grazie*.'

The old man collected the nets under his arms then, with his stooped, painful gait, walked away.

I stepped into the bow of the dinghy, Felix undid the rope from the bollard and took up the oars. We rowed out of the bay, hoisted an amber sail and drifted with the breeze to where the rugged landscape unfurled — our first view of a Mediterranean coastline from the sea. I don't remember how long we sailed in that borrowed dinghy, but when I close my eyes I can still evoke the saffron light, the shimmer on the water, the stone villas clinging to rock, cascades of bright bougainvillea, the dark pines, the sound of sea rolling onto the shore, the scent of summer, the salt air, our stunned silence. By the time we tied up back at the quay, the lights had already come on in the piazza and along the quay. Felix looked at me, then said, 'One day, we'll have a boat and sail the Mediterranean!'

For us, arriving in Portofino many years later was a nostalgic experience. From the sea the coastline was unchanged, and as picturesque as ever. But on shore it was more crowded and noisier than in 1953. We thought of our old fisherman, and wondered what had happened to him. We looked into restaurants, at people along the esplanade, and felt our age. The quay was filled with sleek yachts and cruisers. As we motored in, a cruiser pulled out and the *ormeggiatore* let us tie up.

An *ormeggiatore* is an Italian institution. He reigns supreme over the public wharves and quays by holding the key to the water taps. To tie up in public ports you need his approval (unless he happens to be at home for siesta, in which case you sneak in).

Having a berth on the quay made it easy for us to go ashore for the celebratory meal we had promised ourselves. And a celebratory meal in Portofino is no flippant matter.

We thanked our kind *ormeggiatore* by asking him to top up our water tank, in spite of the fact that we'd filled it the previous day in Lerici. Those few litres were a sufficient excuse for a hefty tip.

We booked a table on a terrace overlooking the bay and ordered the *specialita della casa*, the specialty of the house — *branzino* (bass) baked in 2 kg of sea salt.

'I think we had half a pizza each in 1953,' I reminisced.

'We've travelled a long way since then.'

Overwhelmed by the occasion, the awareness of our good fortune, and the knowledge that our time was limited, I clutched Felix's hand.

The following morning we motored to Paraggi, a bay adjoining Portofino, put down anchor in 12 m of water and had a late breakfast. A breeze had dispersed the summer haze and filled the bay with the scent of pines, the water was like velvet. Above us a gull was gliding in an updraft. High on the hill, cascades of burgundy bougainvilleas spilled over the Hotel Splendido's terraced gardens. It was early, and few people were about.

By lunchtime, a group of teenagers in hired rowing boats were diving into the sparkling water. Guests in large hats trudged from the Hotel Splendido down a donkey trail to the water, while up on the hill, white-gloved waiters served more guests at tables set under foliage. A short distance out at sea, a parade of luxury yachts was in progress. On the decks beer-bellied men in garish shorts strutted alongside tall, and occasionally bare-topped, girls. Waiters in black trousers, white jackets and bow ties dispensed drinks.

By sunset everyone had disappeared and we were alone in the bay. It was a bright night, lights glowed around the shore, the water rippled like coloured silk, cicadas trilled, fireflies flickered and the scent of late summer warmed the air. I thought, 'We'll remember today as clearly as the day we hoisted the old fisherman's sail.'

Our lives had taken on a routine and we were happy in the stability of our cocoon. We bought the paper when we were ashore, listened to the BBC news and tuned into the Livorno weather report at least three times a day. '*Chiamata generale, chiamata generale, chiamata generale, Livorno radio, per il servizio bulletino del meteo…*' We no longer needed to wait for the English translation.

We read a lot, especially books on Tuscany. I was so engrossed in J. H. Plumb's *The Pelican Book of the Renaissance,* I didn't want to finish it. 'You know,' I said to Felix, 'pot-latching, conspicuous consumption, riotous living, nepotism, scandalous behaviour, pursuit of power, were all there in the fifteenth and sixteenth centuries. It was an integral part of life in the city states in Central Italy. Although most Popes' lives were not exactly virtuous, at least they had the good sense to employ people like Michelangelo and Raphael.' I raved on.

The day after we returned to Viareggio, we hired a car and drove to Beaulieu to pick up our Renault. Like a faithful dog, it had waited for us for almost three months. Not only was it filthy, it also had an enormous blob of chewing gum glued to its bonnet. Doubtless this was payback from one of the shop owners whose window display it had obstructed. But as soon as Felix connected the bits he'd disconnected, the faithful animal came to life, purred and revved, and away we went. We were now ready for Tuscany.

'Pisa is only 20 km away, Lucca 27 km, Florence 90 km.' I was on a high.

'But I have to do a few running repairs first.'

Felix's Italian was now almost as good as his French. With a limited number of verbs, nouns and body language thrown in, he was able to discuss the radio with the radio *maestro*, the refrigeration repairs with the refrigeration *supremo*, not to mention be able to ask for everything he needed at the ship chandler and hardware stores. Grammar, agreements, tenses… he decided he'd attend to these some other time. He was teaching me words he'd picked up, such as *pilla* for battery, *frizione* for clutch…And as soon as the latest repairs were done, we were ready.

'First, let's go to Lucca. We've never been there.'

We took the small by-ways to the thick ramparts that girdle Lucca. Along these walls, the dark branches of trees were already discernable as autumn leaves fluttered to the ground. We walked into the old town, with its eleventh century cathedral and peeling gothic palaces, reminders of the city's ancient wealth, and we felt we'd entered a Renaissance world the twentieth century had left untouched. By lunchtime Felix was tired and starved. We found a restaurant and sat under a pergola covered in grape vines.

'What is the specialty in Lucca?' I asked the cheerful, plump woman with a slight limp. She looked as if she'd cooked for a large family all her life.

'Ah, *signora*, in Lucca *tutto è speciale*...everything is special.' If you are hungry, soup, *zuppa di magro* is very good. Also *tortelli casalinghi, cannelloni...*'

We had a long lunch of *zuppa di magro*, a meal in itself, too much wine, and continued to watch the passing parade. 'I need a siesta,' I said, and loosened my belt. 'Time to go home.'

We made our way to our car and found it hemmed in by a car in front, and another behind. We walked around it and wondered what to do. Soon a small crowd gathered.

'*Che maleducazione!* Such rudeness!' An elderly man with a walking stick surveyed the situation. '*Guardate!*...Look at that!' He said to three strapping young men. They took one look at us, waved Felix and me aside, discussed the situation among themselves, and then without much ado, rocked our car up and down, heaved our front bumper bar over the car in front and turned it sufficiently for us to get in.

'*Bravo!*' A roar went up.

'*Grazie tanto.*' We shook hands with everyone, got into the car, waved and made for home. 'There's no end to the advantage of old age...' I muttered.

The weather was noticeably cooler and the days shorter, so we left for Siena at dawn, avoiding the *autostrade* and driving along minor roads into the Tuscan landscape, past picturesque villages on mountain peaks, built not for grand views, but for strategic defence. Feuds and competitions between Florence, Pisa, Lucca and Siena had once been vicious, and frequently led to war.

Every now and then we took breaks to walk in these villages, along meandering lanes into small squares with stone houses, terracotta roofs, green shutters and window boxes. We looked through archways into courtyards where geraniums trailed on weathered walls, and cats warmed themselves.

Towards midday, Felix had a fit of coughing, so we went to a bar to get water. It was a shabby place, as if it had been untouched for years. When the old man behind the counter saw us, he stopped and offered Felix a glass of water. We ordered cappuccinos and sat at a table outside, where an elderly man sat gazing into the distance, a glass of wine in front of him, a cocker spaniel at his feet. He was carefully dressed in a brown hound's-tooth jacket and grey wool trousers. His features were patrician, thin and chiselled. His hair, carefully brushed to one side, was sparse and mottled grey. It was a silent place. Now and again a puff of wind brushed past.

When the old man brought us our coffees, he shuffled past the man at the table and nodded respectfully to him. Felix and I spoke quietly as we inspected a map to work out which route to take. We must have interrupted the man's thoughts, because he turned and smiled. 'You are English?' he asked.

'No, Australian.'

'I was in Australia for some years, a prisoner of war. It was a good place to be.' His English was fluent with a heavy Italian accent.

'I suppose you came back to Italy after the war.'

'Yes, I liked Australia very much, but I had to come back to my family.'

We would have liked to ask more but he seemed a private man, lonely and sad.

'Are there many young people here?' I asked.

'No, this is not a place for young people. They move to the cities, partly for work, partly for the life. They come back to visit their parents or old relatives. Sometimes they come for

RINA HUBER

holidays with their children, to show them what real chickens and cows look like. Here everybody knows everything about everybody, and young people don't like that. They like to move about, to travel. The cities offer them more. These places are dying, unless of course they can be turned into tourist resorts. No one in this village is interested in attracting visitors, that's why it looks so neglected.'

He seemed shrouded in sadness. When the conversation turned to our drive to Siena, he advised us which route to take. We finished our coffee, shook hands and left him to his reminiscences.

It was almost lunchtime when we reached the outskirts of Siena. The twentieth century had encroached on most medieval Italian towns, and parking stations had sprung up in the outskirts. We parked, then walked up a long steep path past young people clutching books as they emerged from a university campus. From the top of a hill we looked across a wide valley towards the rooftops, towers, belfries and ramparts of Siena, bathed in a golden light — 'burnt siena'. We entered a gate and walked down a narrow street. Although the most recent Palio had finished some days earlier, we passed two boys dressed in medieval costumes beating drums.

The Palio, the central event in the life of Siena, has continued uninterrupted for over 700 years. It is a bareback horse race in which each year seven of the seventeen *contrade* or city wards take part. The race entails racing three times round the central, fan-shaped Campo or piazza and lasts about two minutes. As soon as one Palio is over, preparations begin for the next one. The Sienese don't see the Palio as just a sport — it has the features of a ritual and politics as well as those of a game. While the horses are drawn by lot, the *contrade* hire their own jockeys. These are mercenaries who can never be trusted. Although each *contrada* promises their jockey a bonus if he wins, the jockeys also enter into secret agreements with other *contrade*, so the outcome is never predictable and large sums of money are involved.

On the day of the race, the city is decorated with flags and bunting, people hang from windows and climb poles. A deafening cacophony of shouts fills the air, and the smells of horse manure and human sweat permeate the piazza. The winner receives a *palio* or banner, and celebrations continue unabated through the night. Although we had come just days after the most recent Palio, judging by the boys we met, preparation for the next one was already under way.

When we entered the Piazza del Campo, it was a beehive of tourists. The back streets were packed, shops were filled with souvenirs, and countless languages hummed. 'This is like the tower of Babel,' Felix commented. Just then, the bells of the Duomo struck, and from all corners of Siena, churches and basilicas sounded in response. A shudder ran through me as deep sounds beat in unison — boom, boom, boom. A breeze stirred, and a dog cried plaintively. We stood and listened. The sky was already a deep blue, and high above a campanile I glimpsed the white outline of a new moon.

'You know, being a Pope in medieval times was an enviable job, better than being one of today's CEOs. They could do just as they pleased — have women, children, with no media or journalists to print salacious gossip. Take Pope Pius II. He rebuilt the village where he was born, forced his cardinals and dignitaries to buy properties there, and chose a Florentine architect to build the first truly Renaissance town, which was re-named Pienza.'

Felix laughed as I read on.

'When Enea Silvio Piccolomini was born no one could have imagined that he would become a Pope. But in 1458 he was elected Pope Pius II. His early ambition was to re-build the impoverished village where he was born into a summer resort for himself and his court. He hired the Florentine architect Bernardo Rossellino to build what would become the first, perfectly harmonious Renaissance town, Pienza. But the architect had spent three times the original estimate and anticipated punishment. Shaking with fear, he presented himself before the Pope, who addressed him as follows: 'You did well, Bernardo, to lie to us about what this undertaking would cost us. Had you spoken the truth, you would have never persuaded us to spend so much money, and this fair palace, and this church, the loveliest in all Italy would never have existed…We thank you and consider you deserving of special honour.'

Pienza, 50 km from Siena, is a quiet place. As we stood in the square, the only sound was of a young man riding a Lambretta. We walked through the courtyard of the papal palace onto a vast terrace with a view over a valley, the Val d'Orcia, towards Monte Amiata. Only a handful of people stood there, speaking in whispers. Pienza was hushed, as if silent spirits reigned there. Below, the setting sun blazed on scattered windows in the valley, and fleecy clouds raced across the sky.

> Dear Kids,
> This is almost the end of our second summer. Our six weeks in Tuscany have been wonderful. We're leaving the car in Florence with Grazia and Giovanni, and hope to find mail from you there. We'll phone you when we get there. We plan to sail south now and leave *Galatea* on the dry for the winter in a boatshed on the Tiber near Rome. A couple we met in Sardinia keep their boat there and offered to look after her. Then we'll drive back to London via Paris. We'd like

to find a little flat to rent in Paris and spend next winter there instead of London. Wouldn't it be great to have Emma and Jackie with us in Paris for Christmas 1990?

Lots of love, Mum & Dad

◎ ◎ ◎ ◎

We put *Galatea* on the dry using an antique crane belonging to a boatshed on the banks of the Tiber at Fiumare Grande and farewelled her for the winter.

Then we took the train to Florence, picked up the car, drove back to Fiumare Grande, loaded the belongings we needed and drove to Paris. There, we found a flat to rent for the following winter, then made for London. It was a dramatic winter: on 9 November 1989 the Berlin Wall came down.

In London, I had one major priority. During the previous months I'd learnt to live with my hair colour, a melange of apricot pink. But now I was paranoid. I admit that I'd started pulling out grey hairs when I was 8, but the numbers failed me by the time I was 30. It wasn't that I minded getting old. I just didn't fancy myself grey.

But being at sea for months and moving from port to port tested my resolve to stay brown. Every four or five weeks, I went in search of the cleanest looking salon in whichever town or village we happened to find ourselves, and explained, in what I assumed was reasonable French or Italian, that I wanted a medium to dark brown. To confirm this I pointed out the colour on a chart.

Yet time and again I left the salon in horror. It was as if I sported a new wig every few weeks. The final straw occurred when I emerged with a hair colour that was a cross between pink and apricot. I didn't wait for the woman to explain. I fled without paying, and by the time I reached *Galatea* I was in a state of apoplexy.

'That's it! I'm going grey!'

Felix's head and shoulders were deep in the engine's cavity when I stepped on board, and before he'd even extricated himself, he said, 'Hi, how did you go?' No sooner had he uttered this than his face emerged and his jaw dropped. I heard a long 'Ohhhh!' followed by a pained attempt at a laugh. Then, realising that for me this was no laughing matter, he added, 'Honey, don't worry, when we get to London you can get it fixed. What the hell, you can wear your straw hats meanwhile, and you know I don't care.'

'You mightn't care, but I do! And from now on, I'm going grey!'

'You do whatever you like, but you know you won't like being grey.'

So, the day after we arrived back in London, I made straight for Toni & Guy, an upmarket salon near Bond Street. I was in tears as I explained my problem to a young woman called Deborah. From her sympathetic manner, I felt she was accustomed to handling women in distress. Probably most of London's chic and stylish had, at one time or another, passed through the portals of Toni & Guy in a state of shock.

Tall and slim, with an intelligent face and long fair hair, Deborah put a gentle hand on my shoulder and said, 'Don't worry, it's easily fixed. And as for the boat, why don't you tint your own hair?'

'I can't do that. How could I do the back of my head?'

'Ask whoever is on the boat with you to do the back.'

'There's only my husband on the boat.'

'Is he any good with his hands?'

'Not bad, but he wouldn't have a clue how to put on tint.'

'Why don't you get him to come into the salon tomorrow and I'll show him.'

'Are you sure?'

'Of course.' She smiled and passed me a box of tissues.

When I got home I looked at Felix imploringly. 'The girl at Toni & Guy said that if you come in with me tomorrow, she'll show you how to tint hair. Would you mind?' It took him a second to reply, 'Sure, I wouldn't mind. Come the revolution, I can put up a shield on marinas: APPENDIX REMOVED, TEETH EXTRACTED AND HAIR TINTED.'

'You know you drive me crazy with your humour!'

Felix dressed for the occasion. Corduroy trousers, beige polo neck skivvy and a Harris tweed jacket — which, alas, did not have leather elbow patches — and an amused smile.

'This is my husband.' I introduced him to Deborah. 'It's really very good of you,' I said in an embarrassed tone.

'Not at all.' She then turned to Felix. 'Well, let's go downstairs. That's where we do all the tinting.'

A row of women wrapped in pastel gowns, their hair at various stages of tinting and streaking, with clumps of hair wrapped in silver foil, sat peering into magazines. Smooth faces and shaped eyebrows bore the marks of regular facials. Their shoes and handbags were distinctly up-market.

A young girl wrapped a plastic cape over my gown and led me to a chair. Deborah wasted no time. She tied a tinting gown around Felix. 'I hope you're good with your hands. Now I'll show you how to put on these gloves. They're like surgical gloves, quite thin and tear easily...' Felix gave me a fleeting smile in the mirror.

'Now then,' Deborah continued, 'you stir the peroxide with the tint like this...then you part the hair into four segments, put these clips in...' She showed him exactly what to do. Looking into the mirror, I noticed two women, eyebrows raised, convey messages to each other, which I read to be, 'What on earth is a 60-year-old apprentice doing at Toni & Guy?'

When Deborah handed Felix the brush, he looked confident and acted as if he were about to varnish *Galatea*'s rails, which prompted Deborah to say that he showed distinct talent. The women in the mirror looked horrified.

With my hair back to its original brown, I was ecstatic, and Felix was delighted with himself. Deborah proceeded to write down the colour formula and a list of tools we would need. From then on our tinting equipment accompanied us on all our travels.

Dear Kids,

It was wonderful to find a bundle of letters when we arrived in London. So civilised after trying to collect couriered mail in Italy which never arrived. Also a relief to phone you without having to go through Berne Radio.

We feel so lucky to have had a great summer with little drama in spite of our steep learning curve on how not to sink in the Mediterranean. And now that Dad has acquired yet another skill, hair tinting, which has solved my hair problem, we can turn our attention to the wonders of London. Theatres, concerts, exhibitions...we've been busy booking. Our only problem is having to look for a flat to rent each winter, not to mention living in a different place every year. We're toying with the idea of buying a small pad which would make life a lot easier — we shall see.

We're seeing friends and I must say it's a relief to have ordinary English conversations without mentally translating into French and Italian, no matter how much we enjoyed it. Some of our Sydney crowd will be in London during the next few weeks. That's part of the joy of living here. Most people who go overseas seem to pass through London.

I hope you like this selection of photos, we have many more which we'll show you when we come home in February. Of course you can't expect Dad to stay still for too long, so we plan to spend a few days in Paris in the New Year. I've sent off birthday presents for Jackie and Emma, hope they like them. Hope you're all well and not overworked.

Lots of love, from Us Two

In February, our four weeks with the family in Sydney were a break for Felix. No repairs, no need to worry about what could go wrong next. His eyes had improved, and he enjoyed reading for long periods. The fact that he couldn't write by hand didn't worry him — he typed letters and I wrote the envelopes. But after a month he needed to be on the move again.

We left London in March, drove to Germany, and then along Germany's scenic route, the 'Romantic Road' from Wurzburg to Rothenburg and Augsburg. Much of the way was along the Tauber River valley, where willows in the palest of green swayed in the spring breeze in a landscape evocative of medieval times. We drove slowly south, and reached *Galatea* in Rome four weeks later.

chapter five

It had been raining heavily when we arrived at Fiumare Grande, and the place was a sea of mud. We parked the car on a patch of grass and the remains of asphalt. *Galatea* was just as we'd left her, on the dry. Ludovico and Anita, the couple we'd met in Sardinia, had kept an eye on her during the winter months.

The marina was a long boatshed on the banks of the Tiber near Fiumicino. It had a café and an office, whose staff more than made up for the lack of facilities one expects in modern marinas. There was an added attraction. A community of cats and dogs in all shapes and sizes roamed freely, bred at a prodigious rate and were a testament to the nutritious merits of pasta in all stages of decomposition. An antique automatic washing machine was available for the use of clients who were not in a rush. One wash took well over three hours but cost one-fifth of the local laundrette rate. A ten-point list of instructions was stuck on the wall above it, the last of which read: 'It is strictly forbidden to wash live domestic animals in this machine.'

The shower and toilet facilities left much to be desired. But the pleasure of showering with a limitless supply of hot water was irresistible, even though the only clean item in and around the shower was the water itself. 'We can avoid the plague if we make sure we only touch the floor, and wash our feet when we're back on board,' Felix assured me. At night we heard the screeching of rodents, but as we always pulled up the gangplank before we went to bed, we ignored them.

Felix's first crisis was replacing an engine filter. After searching every ship chandler and hardware store around Fiumicino, he contacted his ever reliable Sydney diesel mechanic, Ken Evans, via Berne Radio.

'G'day, Ken.'

'G'day, Felix. Where are ya?'

'Near Rome airport. Sitting on the Tiber, having trouble getting spares for the filter. They don't have Nissan diesels here. What d'ya reckon Ken?'

'Jeez, fancy that! OK, Felix, I'll send ya what ya need tomorrow. Gimme the address and I'll courier it. Should get it to ya in two or three days.'

'Thanks, mate. I'll spell the address for ya...'

Meanwhile, we did a lot of sightseeing in and around Rome. Two and a half weeks after the phone call to Sydney, the filter still hadn't arrived. Subsequent phone calls traced the package to customs in Milan. We were assured that, if we sent 19 000 lire to customs in Milan, we could have the parcel within days. A week later the parcel arrived.

'Geez, it's awfully heavy. I hope he sent the right bit.' Felix looked worried, and unpacked the parcel slowly and carefully. Suddenly, he beamed. 'Look at this, good old Ken! He put in a can of Fosters with the filter. What an Oz thing to do.'

'Here's to Ken's health!' We shared the can of beer.

'Oh, I almost forgot. The boat insurance is due in three weeks. Italian mail is so erratic, we'd better post the cheque express today. You'd better take it to the post office. I can't move just now.' Felix was on the floor, squeezed between the sink and the cracked toilet of the aft cabin, working out how to install the new one.

Clutching the envelope, I set off to the post office.

'If I send this letter express, will it arrive in London in a few days?' I asked the girl behind the desk. She glared as if she'd never heard such a stupid question. An elderly man standing near me turned, and said in a matter of fact way, 'The only way you can make sure a letter leaves Italy is to post it at the Vatican.'

Is he cracking a funny? Am I expected to laugh? I wondered. I was about to ask him whether stamps bought in the Vatican included prayers for quick delivery, but decided against it. Certainly, there was no twinkle in his eye. The girl behind the counter narrowed her eyes, stared first at him, then at me, and spat out, '*He* obviously knows when an express letter will get to London.'

I thanked the man. He nodded. Back at the marina, still clutching the envelope, I asked the girl who ran the office about express mail. She confirmed that if the letter was really important, we should post it at the Vatican. So we drove to the Vatican.

The next time I went to the post office was to buy stamps.

'Stamps?' the girl asked peremptorily.

'Yes, stamps. For England and Australia.'

'But I don't have any stamps!' she replied, as if any fool would know this.

'Well, when will you have more stamps?'

'When they arrive I will have more stamps!'

We also learnt a lot about banks. Not only the hours of opening and closing, but also the different rules. Once we understood the idiosyncrasies of each one, life became tolerable. With only one Eurocheque in my wallet, I ventured into the Banco di Lavoro to cash it. I'd made an unfortunate error with the date — out by one day. I altered and initialled it.

'Are you kidding?' was the expression on the teller's face as he returned it to me.

'But this is the only cheque I have on me,' I begged, 'and our next meal depends on my cashing it.' It was all to no avail. I stormed out in a huff and marched towards another bank, the Banco d'Italia. It was closed. A woman passing by noticed me standing at the closed front door. '*Signora*,' she said, 'there is a *sciopera*, a strike, at this bank, but there's another bank around the corner, it's open.' By now Felix had joined me. We made for the bank the woman suggested. It was called Banco di Santo Spirito.

'Do you think this bank will accept an initialled date?'

'If it has something to do with the Vatican, they'll accept it,' Felix said. 'An initialled date shouldn't worry them too much as long as there's real money at the other end. Give it a go.' I made for the nearest teller. He didn't even bother to look up before he cashed it.

'From now on, we only use the Vatican Post Office and Vatican Banks!'

◎◎◎◎

We were moored close to the excavations of Ostia Antica, ancient Rome's principal port, which dates from the fourth century BC. At its peak, 100 000 people lived there. By the third century AD, the accumulation of silt began the port's decline, and within another 100 years it was abandoned. Extensive excavations revealed a complex, sophisticated town with merchants' guilds and trading links throughout the known world. We walked along the main streets where the furrows of carriage wheels are still visible, down side streets and through shopping arcades where mosaics at the entrances to shops advertised their wares. Bars and bath houses, theatres, temples, synagogues, shipping offices, food shops, public latrines, warehouses, even an erotica palace — Ostia Antica had them all.

With a little imagination we could smell, see and hear the multitudes of people on the streets — shopping, eating, conducting business and enjoying themselves.

'Let's go one more time to visit Ostia,' Felix suggested, a couple of days before we intended to leave the mainland. Unlike previous occasions when we'd been there, the place was packed with tour buses. In fact, it was so crowded we decided to turn back to the car, and found the back window broken and Felix's jacket stolen. We spent the rest of the day driving around Rome to get the window fixed, which was easier than getting stamps at the post office. In all our years of travelling, this was the only time that our car was broken into — and on this occasion we'd left it for less than half an hour.

During our seven weeks on the Tiber, we'd come to know Rome and its surroundings well, but it was time to move on. On the way to Florence, where we intended to leave our car with friends, we spent time in Umbria, and found it so beautiful we decided to rent a house and have a family get-together there one day.

'Let's make it our 50th wedding anniversary. May 1999!'

'Funny how we go on making plans,' I thought. 'We never speak about the bad times that await us, but that's how we cope, that's how I cope, and Felix knows it.'

> Hi Kids,
> We're almost off. We did a lot of sightseeing, Ostia Antica, Tivoli, Villa Adriana, Tarquinia, which has hundreds of Etruscan tombs, and of course Rome. We left the car again with Grazia and Giovanni in Florence, but managed to spend time in Assisi,

Spoleto, Perugia, Orvieto, Todi and Gubbio on the way, and took the train back to Rome from Florence.

Dad's well, although he's been getting tired.

He maintains that the most useful thing he has ever done is to work with a mechanic one school holiday, a plumber another year, and then an electrician. The next most useful is abdominal surgery, which has taught him to work in the dark by 'feeling'. Well, he's been doing a lot of that on the boat.

You'll gather that we haven't had much reading time lately, but we've seen a lot of Italy. We have, however, re-read large bits of Homer. The reason for this urgent re-reading is that we'll now be covering Odysseus's route — that is, the Aeolian Islands and the Strait of Messina, reputed to be the original Scylla and Charybdis, which you will doubtless remember from your Greek mythology.

I'll post this today and with luck you should get it in under two months. We'll try and phone next week, depending on where we find ourselves. We're sorry to leave Italy, but looking forward to the Dalmatian Coast.

Keep well, lots of love, M & D

◎◎◎◎

The mist was thick as we set sail for the Pontine Islands the following morning. These were very much part of the Ancient Roman world. The harbour entrance to Ventotene, the most interesting of the islands, is barely 15 m across. It was originally a Roman galley harbour carved out of volcanic rock. For the Romans, this was a prison that once held notables such as

Julia, daughter of Augustus, Octavia, the wife of Nero, and others. In more recent times, Mussolini used Ventotene as a penal settlement for political prisoners. We stayed for a couple of days. On the third day, Felix looked up at the sky and announced, 'It's going to be a brilliant day. Your turn to read.' Since our collision off Corsica, we were strict about taking turns to read when we were out at sea — two hours on, two hours off.

We manoeuvred out of Ventotene soon after sunrise, and with all sails drawing, we hoped to cover the 22 miles to Ischia by lunchtime. The 9.30 forecast, however, was for a *burasca*, gale.

'Better turn on the engine and get there before it really starts to blow.'

While I went down to fasten everything that was lying loose, Felix shortened the headsail, took down the main and increased the throttle. We were making 7 knots and arrived at the entrance to Ischia harbour just as the gale hit. We were not the only ones making it into port. Ferries, hydrofoils, motor boats, yachts, fishing vessels — everything afloat within a visible radius — was negotiating the narrow entrance to the shelter of Porto d'Ischia. We radioed the harbour authorities for permission to enter. But that was purely academic.

'You don't expect a response, do you? We're in Italy.'

'Let's make for any free spot along the public quay before the others get ahead of us.' Felix was racing the other boats. We made for the nearest spot. The *ormeggiatore*, his arms in full flight, belly shuddering, face growling, spat out: '*Via! Via!* Go! Go!' It was clear he wouldn't let us in. Felix reversed and made for another spot. The *ormeggiatore* followed us. Gesticulating with every part of his body, he was sending us a message — '…it would be unhealthy for you to tie up!'

'For God's sake, let's get away from here. If we go ashore, he'll sink her!' I shouted.

'Bastard! We're legally entitled to tie up to a public quay!' Felix had lost his cool and I was scared.

Then, with the engine at full throttle, and cursing the *ormeggiatore,* he reversed with such force it sounded as if the gearbox had fallen apart. The dinghy, which was tied to the stern rail, caught a mooring line and capsized, the outboard was in the air. Felix let go of the wheel, and as we both rushed to grab the rope that was still tied to the aft rail, the helm spun free, and *Galatea* collided with boats on both sides. A large vessel was already waiting to pull into the spot we were vacating. As we struggled to pull the dinghy in closer, *Galatea* drifted out into the heaving waves, bumping into everything in her path.

'Take the helm!' Felix yelled. I took the wheel, swerved *Galatea* to port, then starboard, with craft on all sides.

'Let go the rope and let's get out of here!' I shrieked over the blazing *burasca.* Then, as I turned to Felix for instructions, I realised he wasn't there. For a flash I thought he'd gone overboard, but just as I was about to panic, I caught sight of his feet clinging to the gunwale. The *ormeggiatore* chose this moment to fire a litany of curses. He made it quite clear that we were to 'fuck off'. I didn't see Felix right the dinghy, but I did hear him yell, 'OK, turn and get out of here!'

Ignoring all who were after our blood, we made a dash for Procida, Ischia's ugly sister, a couple of miles away, where we detected a ship that looked as if it had lain abandoned there since Armistice Day, 1945. Without asking anyone for anything, we tied up to it.

We sat in silence and stared at motorbikes tearing up and down the quay, and turned our backs on yet another *ormeggiatore* who glared at us. We were both in a foul mood.

After giving himself time to cool off, Felix approached the outboard motor. 'The bloody thing's buggered. I can't get it to start!' He tried cursing in English, to no avail, then he poured himself a large whisky and sat for a long time. Later, reverting to his usual patient self, he started to take it apart. He washed all the components in fresh water, dried them and put them together again.

'I'll give it another go.' He pulled the starter belt. The motor spat, gurgled, then purred.

'Well, that's that!' Felix stretched out on a bunk, closed his eyes and went to sleep.

The following morning we pretended the previous day had never happened. Our only concession to the events of the day before was an agreement that *ormeggiatori* (apart from the one in Portofino) were a nasty lot, and that we wouldn't discuss them again.

'Let's have a big Oz breakfast, stay downstairs and pretend we're home.' Oz breakfasts of bacon and eggs, toast, marmalade and coffee were our cure for most things. If we also stayed in the saloon, we could pretend we were in Broken Bay, near our favourite tree at Smith's Creek, with a kookaburra on the crosstrees.

The smell of sizzling bacon and eggs and the aroma of fresh coffee and slightly burnt toast filled the saloon.

'OK, so what do we do next?' I said.

'There's a fellow I read about in one of the yachting journals who now lives on Ischia. His name's Steve Evans. He used to sail for many years, but he's now decided to become a landlubber. They say he likes to talk to yachties passing through. We can get the ferry from here to Ischia, and see if we can look him up in the phone book.'

Steve and his partner were at home when we phoned, and invited us to their place. They were very friendly, and we learnt a great deal from them — for instance, about the *modus operandi* of the quays in Ischia. Apparently we were chased out because the local Mafia controlled the quays there, and only Neapolitan clients who paid were allowed to tie up. Steve also gave us a lot of advice on sailing the waters of southern Italy, including a warning about the horrors of being caught in a gale in the unsheltered waters of the Golfo di Squillace, the Gulf of Squalls.

'When it blows there, it really blows hard. I've been through it twice, and let me tell you, I wouldn't want to be caught there again.' He also suggested where we should go and what we should see. 'The Riace Warriors at the Museum in Reggio Calabria, and...you're going to Capri, of course.'

'Well, we weren't sure, especially after our experience yesterday. We have this dread of beautiful people in Gucci sunglasses...'

'Capri is too beautiful to miss,' he said. 'True, it's very, very expensive to tie up there, but it's worth it. This is the best time of the year to see it. Capri in May is at its most beautiful. I'm sure you won't regret it.'

It was May, and how right he was! Early next morning we set sail.

I always marvelled when, having plotted a course and set the autohelm to it, our destination appeared first on the radar, and then imperceptibly through the haze and mist to the naked eye. There is something majestic about an island rising from the sea.

As we neared Capri, its distant grey came alive with blues, greens and tinges of orange where the sun reflected off the sheer cliff face. All around the island, clouds of gulls soared in the spring sky. Below, a fleet of multicoloured butterfly sails fluttered in the breeze as an array of large yachts paraded in review.

'Shall we radio for permission to enter?' I asked.

'They're unlikely to answer, so there's not much to lose.'

'What if they don't let us tie up, like in Ischia?'

'We need to think of a way to outsmart them.' We sat and thought.

'I know, let's tell them I'm very sick!' I said.

'What makes you think they'd care?'

'Italians melt when someone's sick. Especially a mother. A wife is a wife, you can always get another one. But a mother, well, you can only have one.'

'Do you want me to say you're my mother?'

'Don't you dare. I'd clobber you one if you did!'

'OK, let's try my wife is very sick, *mia moglie è molto malata*, how's that?'

'*Perfetto*, what shall I be suffering from? A bad heart would be OK.'

'Right, so here goes.' Felix went down, turned on the radio, took a deep breath and started, 'Radio Capri, Radio Capri, this is *Galatea*, Golf Alfa Lima Alfa Tango Echo Alfa, requesting permission to enter harbour.'

We were shocked — an instant reply. '*Galatea, Galatea, qui radio Capri, è impossibile entrare.*'

'Shit, what now?' For some seconds Felix was stunned, but then continued, 'Radio Capri, Radio Capri, *qui* Galatea, *mia moglie è molto malata*.' Long silence.

'Galatea, Galatea, *un momento*.' It was a very long *momento*. Then, 'Galatea, Galatea, *entrate*, we will send somebody to help you.'

'*Grazie*, Radio Capri...'

'Now you'd better start looking sick!'

We felt proper frauds as the Capri tender met us at the entrance and guided us to a spot along the quay. They took our lines and helped Felix tie up. The harbour was crowded with boats participating in a regatta. Crowds were milling on shore and along the quay. When I attempted to help tie up, Felix pushed me down. 'For Chrissake stay down and look crook.'

I heard him explain that I had a *mal di cuore*. It was my heart.

'I'm surprised they didn't bring a doctor and a priest,' I whispered as they left.

On one side of us was a small boat flying an American pennant. The fellow on board spoke fluent Italian.

'Excuse me, but where does one go to pay?' Felix asked.

'Pay, pay?' he replied in a stunned Brooklyn accent. 'I never pay, I just play at being dumb.' We introduced ourselves. Bruno was a laid-back navigator, sailing round the world in the kind of boat where prayers would not go amiss. I wondered which junkyard he'd bought it from.

'Did they just let you come in? What about the *ormeggiatore*?'

'I never look them in the face. It's a technique I've learnt.'

Felix and I looked at each other and shrugged. When Bruno looked bored with ingenues such as us, we turned to the English couple on the 18-m (55-ft) ketch flying a Hong Kong flag on the other side.

'Excuse me,' Felix started, 'could you tell me where the marine office is to pay?'

'Oh...' the man replied, 'we never pay. Well, not until they come up and ask us to pay. They haven't come yet.'

'Don't they come after you as soon as you enter the harbour?'

'Oh, we never ask for permission to enter, we just go in and berth wherever there's a suitable spot. Sometimes we put down an anchor in the middle of the harbour if there's room. Occasionally we have problems with *ormeggiatori*, but otherwise we say nothing and keep a low profile...admittedly, with a boat this size it isn't always easy. Still, one tries.'

We spent an informative afternoon with the Smithards. They gave us all kinds of useful tips on how to get by. 'Above all, try to look dumb and innocent. Play hard at being silly foreigners. Italians will forgive you most things if you do that. Admittedly, some get a little suspicious when they see a boat as big as ours. But on the whole, we get by.'

After several long drinks, we thanked Tom and Jean, and wished them good sailing. They were leaving for the Balearics the following morning.

Given the fraudulent way we'd entered the harbour, it seemed wise for me to stay on board until I could afford to look healthier, so we decided not to go to the village that afternoon. Early next morning, however, we couldn't contain our excitement and boarded the funicular, the tiny train used to ascend the island's precipitous rock face to the village at the top. On both sides of the tracks, houses suspended at the edge of the rock face defied gravity. Small vineyards and other vegetation surrounded houses, clusters of unripe grapes and creepers hung from pergolas. Tiny groves of citrus trees were in bloom. Flowers nuzzled under rocks and between crevices. Geraniums, daisies, poppies, anemones and buttercups faced the sun and swayed in the breeze. We breathed in the scent of jasmine and wisteria curling up trellises, pergolas and stone arches.

From the peak of the funicular, we gazed down the sheer cliffs to the marina and the deep blue water below. 'Hey, look! There's *Galatea*!' The air was thick with birds hang-gliding in slow motion, round and round, tending nests and newborn chicks.

Narrow alleys radiated from the main piazza, there was a buzz of activity everywhere. Hotel porters puffed and pushed luggage on two-wheeled carts. Tourists filled cafés and promenaded past shop windows.

'I've never felt such a fraud in my life,' I said.

'I know what you mean. At least we're plagued by guilt. In any case, perhaps someone from the marina office will come and ask us to pay.' But nobody came.

'Maybe we're on a public marina that's free?' I suggested.

'Are you going to ask?'

'No.'

By the third day we had acclimatised to our luck, and felt perfectly relaxed.

'Let's stay till the end of the week and have a wedding anniversary dinner.'

'Good idea! Meanwhile, let's visit Anacapri.'

The bus ride to Anacapri at the peak of the island was terrifying. As the overloaded bus swayed and lurched at hairpin bends, avoiding oncoming traffic on one side and the vertical precipice on the other, tourists craned and stretched from one side of the bus to the other, rapturously applauding each new vista.

'*Ach, Alfred, kuck doch, wie herrlich!* Look, how fabulous!'

'Harry, did you get that shot?'

'*Mon Dieu, comment c'est magnifique!*'

By the time we reached the top I felt like jelly, and had lost interest in the pilgrimage to Axel Munthe's house, Villa San Michele. 'If we ever come up here again, it'll be on a mule.'

History records that the Emperor Augustus had done a deal with the Neapolitans and exchanged Ischia for Capri in order to build a pleasure garden. However, he died after living on the island for only four years, and the Emperor Tiberius inherited Capri. Tiberius also spent his last years there but like most Roman emperors, he was paranoid about being murdered. And for good reason. To improve his odds of survival, he built twelve villas and lived in a different one each month. But this did not deter his murderer.

We climbed the steep path that leads to the largest of these villas, Villa Jovis. A haunting silence surrounded it. Clusters of wild flowers burst through crevices, under pebbles, between rocks and ruins. Lizards scrambled in and out of cracks, bees droned among the blooms and pines swayed in the breeze. From the peak of the island and from Monte Solaro, the view is still much as Tiberius saw it — spectacular. On most days pollution and haze lingered over the Bay of Naples, the Amalfi coast and the mainland, but the day we were there, the nor'westerly had cleared the air and Naples, its harbour and the coastline glowed in the afternoon sun.

'Whatever you do, think long and hard before sailing into Naples and leaving your boat unattended,' a number of sailing aficionados had warned us. As we had no problem leaving *Galatea* on the marina in Capri, we took the ferry to Sorrento and made our way from there by train to Herculaneum, and by bus to Amalfi and Ravello.

Like Pompeii, Herculaneum was devastated by the eruption of Vesuvius in AD 79, then lay buried until it was accidentally discovered in 1719. We wandered through its neatly excavated streets, the multistoried houses of commoners and patricians, wine-shops, baths, schools and places of worship, and admired the paintings, decorations and mosaics. Unlike Pompeii, Herculaneum was small enough for us to imagine what life must have been like 2000 years ago.

Our magical week in Capri culminated in a gastronomic extravaganza at Il Gattino on our wedding anniversary. We drank toasts to the Emperor Augustus for his fine choice of island, to Steve for persuading us to visit Capri, and to our steep upward learning curve and fraudulent entry into the marina.

◎◎◎◎

When we sailed out of Capri in the early morning, the air was tinged with blue. Following us, a flotilla of boats with multi-coloured sails made its way to a starting line. It was as though we were part of the racing fleet in Sydney. My eyes grew moist and I couldn't bear to look back.

We hoisted sail and set an 80-degree course to take us towards the Amalfi Coast. We planned to sail as far as the promontory before Salerno, then turn south to Agropoli. A light nor'westerly swept *Galatea* towards the Gulf of Salerno, while we sat on the aft deck in the morning sun and watched the bubbling froth spill astern. Ahead, the Amalfi coastline unfolded through the mist. *Galatea*'s sails glistened in the morning sun, crystal ripples cascaded from her bow as she cut through the water, and a benevolent breeze swept past us. All around us was space. Limitless, luminous space and an overwhelming sense of freedom.

In the corner of the cockpit our pot of basil looked happy and released a cloud of scent whenever we touched it. The geranium, tied to the foot of the mizzen, looked a little battered but we hoped our tender care would resuscitate it. Tomatoes strung on their stalks swung on a hook in the galley. Two baskets with lemons, peaches and apricots still moist with dew slid around the floor of the saloon.

'Great forecast,' Felix announced as he climbed into the cockpit bearing a flask of chianti, olives and crackers.

◎ ◎ ◎ ◎

How different a coastline looks from the sea! From a bus the serpentine road — with its twists and turns, jagged rocks, deep gorges, houses stacked precipitously on top of one another and the crystal sea below — is breathtaking, but only a half view. To sail along the coast is to experience the exhilarating whole. Shapes and colours unravel, puffs of air blow the scent from orange and lemon groves out to sea, the sounds of birds echo on the water, seagulls soar above the sails, fish catapult in and out of the sea. From a boat the landscape is a slow, unfolding portrait.

As we passed Punta Campanella, pastel houses suspended in mid-air appeared woven through the landscape, terraces bright with creepers faced the sea. Pines, olive trees and vegetation hugged steep slopes. Below, the sea rolled onto miniscule beaches and sleepy fishing villages nestled against rocks. Blue, red, yellow and green rowing boats, tied to rocks, lapped close to one another and swung from side to side like playing puppies. We passed Positano and hugged the coast to Amalfi. Ravello gazed down to the sea.

'Time for lunch!' Tomatoes grown on board, basil, fetta and olives, a touch of olive oil, a glass of chianti, a stick of ciabatta, peaches, coffee and amaretti Capresi.

At Capo d'Orso we changed course and made for Agropoli.

We sailed into Agropoli's near empty harbour in the late afternoon and tied up to the long new pier. Three small boats were riding at anchor in the bay. Apart from seagulls lazing in an updraft and occasionally squawking, the only sounds were of our sails coming down. Not a soul in sight.

'Must be siesta time. Or maybe time to get ready for the *passeggiata*,' Felix suggested.

We folded the mizzen, stood on the aft deck and looked around. The old town sat fortress-like above the bay. Small square white boxes dotted the stony hillside. Windows glowed red and orange in the setting sun. A steep road led up to the town from the harbour below.

It had been a long day, too full to do anything more than sit with a drink and watch the sunset and the passing parade.

This began with well groomed young men manoeuvring their motorbikes slowly up and down the pier. As the evening progressed, more joined the slow procession. Like strutting peacocks, the young men displayed their plumage — neat jeans, blow-dried hair lacquered into place, dark sunglasses and a powerful grip on polished handlebars. What communication there may have been between them was conveyed with body language. Only an occasional revving punctuated the silence.

'This must be some kind of ritual,' I said.

As the evening progressed, young girls appeared. Long hair, tight miniskirts, high heels, sunglasses judiciously balanced on their heads. The gait was a studied slow motion with a sideways hip swing. Each girl made a brief appearance on the pier, then stepped up onto its protecting wall where she assumed a nonchalant air — with one hand on a swung-out hip, she affected an intense interest in the sky.

The young men continued their slow parade up and down the mole, but now they inspected the miniskirted offerings posing on the high wall above it. As the sky darkened, they peeled off their sunglasses and displayed them in their left breast pockets.

Suddenly a horn blasted, almost catapulting me into the water. A challenge was on. 'This must be a mating ritual. The old piazzas may be too cramped for motorcycles, and there aren't any parents here.'

'The tooting must be a signal. Look at the change in the girls!'

As the air filled with the sound of horns, the girls abandoned their interest in the sky and replaced it with an unashamed interest in the offerings below. A swift nod, a gesture, a glance exchanged in silence secured an agreement. The girl then stepped quickly down the stairs, swung onto the machine, wound her arms around the young man, and off they roared to join the parade of the paired. They continued up and down the mole.

Some time later, a slow-moving trail of cars appeared.

'What's this? Parents? Bet it's the girls' parents.'

In each of the vehicles sat a concerned middle-aged couple. While the father negotiated the car along the quay, the mother craned her neck out the window in a frantic search for her daughter. As soon as she spotted her, she waved and called, '*Angelina!...Angelina!...Ciao!...Ciao!...Angelina!...Ciao!*'

'*Ciao...Mamma. Ciao!*' came the response.

The mother relaxed and sat back in her seat and smiled. No further warning needed. She turned to her husband and pointed out this pair and that.

'She's making a quick assessment of where her daughter's partner ranks in the eligibility stakes,' I suggested. 'This is more than just a *passeggiata*, it's courtship. Modern Agropoli's variation on a Jane Austen ball. A mother's concern for her daughter's reputation and a good match. *Famiglia ed Onore!*'

'You'd need to be an acrobat to do it on a bike, I'd prefer a clapped out car.'

'Oh, you'll never understand the importance of machismo, or the importance of *fare la bella figura*.'

The noise and action continued for much of the night. Gradually the cars thinned, and the motorbikes took off.

We were far from brimming with energy the following morning when we made our way into town to ask about buses to Paestum, an archaeological site we'd been told not to miss.

'*Mi dispiace, non lo so...*Sorry, I don't know,' was everyone's reply. If locals don't know about a bus to Paestum, who does, we wondered.

Mating rituals had kept us awake most of the night and we were tired, ready to give up, when an old lady lugging two shopping bags heard us ask about buses to Paestum and said, 'I'll show you where to get the bus to Paestum. It's not here.'

We followed that gentle, big-bosomed woman as she trundled on heavy legs up the steep hill. We waited at the traffic lights to cross the road. When they turned green, I stepped off the curb, heard a sudden 'swoosh', saw something black flash past, and felt someone grab my arm and jerk me back onto the footpath. The old woman had saved me from a messy encounter with a super-charged motorbike.

'*Signora,*' she said, looking shocked, '*in Italia semaferi sono soltanto un consiglio.* In Italy, traffic lights are only an advice, a suggestion.'

That dear woman took us to the Paestum bus stop, wished us a good day and then went on her way.

After a long wait at the bus stop, we finally got to Paestum. It is one of the most important archaeological sites in Italy, a settlement that had been founded by Greek colonists around 600 BC, and discovered accidentally in 1750. We walked around the impressive excavations. The museum contains many artefacts and remarkable examples of Greek funerary art. The most famous, known as the Diver's Tomb, is box-shaped, with Greek frescoes dating from around 480 BC. We were too weary to see as much as we would have liked, and we were also anxious to get back to *Galatea*.

'I'm beat. All I want is to sleep for 24 hours.'

'OK, let's move out to somewhere quiet,' Felix said.

We untied the lines, motored to the middle of the bay and put down an anchor. But the tooting and hooting of the mating rituals continued relentlessly much of the night. In the morning we were eager to move on.

The only information in the *Italian Waters Pilot* about Scario in the Gulf of Policastro was: '…a small fishing harbour is being built here. Depths and the final form are unknown to date'.

It looked attractive. Pastel houses and date palms lined the harbour front, and scattered on the slopes of a steep mountain were villas, hidden behind tall trees and other vegetation. As we entered the small port, the bells of the pink church at the entrance chimed, an onshore breeze stirred the palms and ragged clouds hung over the hills.

We were the only foreign boat in the harbour. Four fishing boats were tied up along the sea wall, and a number of fishermen sat mending nets. As the afternoon progressed, people dressed for the *passeggiata* strolled along the quay, looked us over and greeted us with '*Buona sera*'.

Meanwhile the fishermen had started to move off to lay their tunny nets. They waved as they passed, and we waved back. When the last boat had left the harbour, we had soup and slumped into bed. In the morning we woke just as the fishing fleet motored in with the night's catch, clouds of seagulls in tow.

While we were breakfasting in the cockpit, a young fisherman stopped to introduce himself. 'I'm Eddo, I work on my father's fishing boat...Can I come on board?'

'Sure, come on, would you like a coffee?'

Eddo looked bright, curious, energetic and, like most of the young generation of fishermen, more gregarious, as well as less inhibited with foreigners than the older generation. 'I hope you don't leave today. We're going to have a sirocco, it lasts three days. Good to stay in port.'

We listened to the weather report and decided to stay. Later that day, Eddo brought his father Pasquale to meet us. They started by calling Felix 'Signor Felice'. A day later, this evolved to a simple 'Felice'. They never tried to call me anything. In fact, as far as they were concerned, I hardly existed.

Eddo loved to come and talk. Sometimes he'd stand on the pier next to the boat and call, 'Felice, Felice!' If I popped my head out to tell him that Felice wasn't on board, he'd leave a message to ask Felice to come and talk to the men under the big tree near the water tap. That was the meeting place where all the elderly and retired returnees from abroad sat for hours chatting. The fishermen joined them when they finished work. It was strictly men only.

On the second morning I asked a wizened, black-clad woman, '*Dov'è il panificio*? Where's the bakery?'

'Ah,' she said, '*è già chiuso*, it's already closed. *Ma venga, venga,* come, come with me, I'll take you to the baker's wife, she'll give you some bread. I'm her mother's cousin.'

We climbed countless stairs and walked past whitewashed houses and pots of geraniums, daisies and bougainvillea to the end of the street.

She stopped in front of a blue door, gave it a few hard bangs and shouted: 'Angelica, Angelica!'

A young woman in high heels and long black hair opened the door. '*Ah, Maria, come stai?* How are you?'

'*Bene, bene*, this *signora* would like some bread.' My good samaritan went on to explain that I was from the English boat that came in the day before. Angelica said she didn't have any bread left. She only had her own loaf. But that didn't deter Maria, her first cousin once removed. '*Allora*, well then,' she said, 'give her yours.'

Angelica looked embarrassed, then grudgingly went to the sideboard, pulled out her loaf and offered it to me. I held out money, but she said, 'No, no, this is my bread so there's nothing to pay.'

No matter how much I protested, she continued to say, 'No, no, I can't take it.' And both Maria and Angelica insisted that I must have the bread. In the end I thought I'd offend them if I didn't take it, so I said, '*Grazie, grazie tanto.*'

The forms of hospitality are varied and have many agendas. As we walked back down the stairs, Maria told me that she had a restaurant up on the hill. 'You know, my husband is a very good cook. Especially fish…' With the bread episode, Maria and I had established a bond. We now 'owed' each other.

'We should eat at Maria's restaurant tomorrow,' I said to Felix as I stepped on board with the bread. 'Yes, of course we must.'

The following night we did. Maria's husband served us the freshest of everything and made us feel special.

It was almost 1 o'clock when I saw Felix ambling along the quay one day. He seemed to have acquired the gait of the old men. The general assembly must have disbanded for lunch. He'd been gone since 11, chatting with the men at their regular meeting spot — under the big tree near the water tap. Between 1 and

5 o'clock everyone was home; not even a dog was allowed to bark.

'What do you all talk about?' I asked.

'It's interesting. A couple of them speak English. They've spent years working in America, but have come back home to retire. Another one used to work in North Africa laying pipelines for an Italian oil company. He speaks French. The fellow from South America speaks Spanish. There are quite a few returnees. They sit there for hours discussing the world, and how it used to be when they worked abroad. With the savings they bring back, they enjoy life here. The fishermen join in when they're not busy.

'They laugh about how everyone is related to everyone else, and that everyone knows everything about everyone else, or at least makes it their business to find out. Most live down near the water. Only the "gentry" live up on the hill. It seems that the higher up the hill you live, the more "up-market" you are. They all love living here, but worry about the proposed building of a road from Naples to Scario. They certainly hope it never gets built. They don't want the "riff raff from Naples" or, for that matter, tourists to come here. No one mentions the Mafia.

'They ask a lot about Australia, and how we like Italy...the food, the wine...

'The fishermen reckon we're in for bad weather, and said we shouldn't leave until it's over. First, they said we'll get a sirocco and then a *ponente,* westerly. They can tell by the clouds over the mountain.'

Eddo and his father Pasquale took Felix under their wing. They came at least twice a day to see if we needed anything. Eduardo, whom we'd met soon after we'd arrived, came down after every weather forecast to keep us up with the latest. He and his wife lived in Milan, but they had a holiday home up on the hill — where the gentry lived. He had held a senior position in the public service before his retirement, but was now a frustrated sailor who'd had to sell his boat to appease his wife. He used any excuse to visit us. After several days of strong winds, which kept us in harbour, he came to tell us that the forecast was for abating winds. We didn't tell him we'd already heard the same report.

'You're going to have a terrific crossing,' he said, almost in tears. He would have loved to have come with us to Lipari, but his wife put her foot down in no uncertain manner.

We fell in love with Scario and its people, but after a week it was time to move on.

The clouds that had hovered over the mountain peak behind Scario during the previous days had lifted, and the fishermen also prepared to leave later that afternoon. It was a perfect day. At 3 o'clock the old men, Eduardo, Eddo, his father and the fishermen watched as we cast off and waved farewell. We expected to reach Lipari the following morning.

For us the start of a passage had a special quality, which was different from sailing along a coast. With an overnight crossing there was a kind of settling into a routine. Even if we didn't expect it to be rough, we were always prepared. The evening before, we checked through our long list in case it did get rough. Before leaving we made everything fast, we filled a thermos with boiling water for tea, prepared bland sandwiches, entered the log, checked the satnav and the radar, coiled the ropes, collected the fenders, stowed everything away and, finally, put on our safety harnesses.

As we motored out of Scario, light clouds dotted the sky, and the diffuse Mediterranean haze permeated the atmosphere. We hoisted sail as soon as we had cleared the bay. The breeze carried us along as we watched Scario with its pink church fade into the distance. I was always apprehensive at the start of a crossing, and relieved when we approached our destination.

My favourite watch was from 2 to 6 in the morning, when the breeze and the sea were gentle, splashes of stars brightened the sky, the moon threw a wide beam onto the water and silver ripples pirouetted in its light. That was when an extraordinary sense of wellbeing and good fortune overwhelmed me. Then, as the night progressed and the strip of dark grey on the eastern horizon began to turn into the palest of pink, I loved to watch the night's gradual change to day.

If we were on deck together, there was little need to speak. We read each other's moods and thoughts. We loved the many different kinds of silence. The silence of a steady wind singing in the shrouds, the constant hiss of *Galatea*'s bow moving through the water, the silence and solitude of a rising dawn, the changing colours of the sea and sky, the scent of the early morning. No matter how familiar, the experience was always different and miraculous. That was when we, a speck adrift on the ocean, became part of all that was around us.

We watched the hills behind Scario fade. A long way ahead, and out of sight, was our destination, the Aeolian islands.

Sailors have always feared the crossing to these islands. The islands' name derived from Aeoleus, the god of winds. Wishing Odysseus a good passage, Aeoleus presented him with a leather bag in which he had tied up all the contrary winds. Odysseus's snooping crew, however, convinced that it was full of treasure, couldn't wait to see what was in the bag. So, when they assumed they were near Ithaca, they opened it. Instead of treasure, out flew all the winds, which then blew them away from their destination. But at the start of our crossing on *Galatea*, it seemed that Aeoleus still had all the winds tied securely in his bag.

When we left port, our immediate concern was the tuna nets that fishermen set and scatter along this coastline. These were a major hazard. To sail into one and then try to untangle the net from the propeller would have been a nightmare. Kerosene flares are supposed to mark each net at regular intervals, but if the sea is rough, they are difficult to see. So we sat sipping tea, on the lookout for nets. The breeze felt cool on our faces, and we listened to the silence. It was strange how, when we were at sea, *Galatea* assumed a life of her own, revelling in the waves and the challenge, responding to the faintest touch on the wheel. While her features changed with the mood of the wind and the sea, the saloon below retained a constancy, the familiar stability of warmth and home.

As the afternoon progressed, Felix looked at the sky. 'I don't like the look of those clouds. Let's reef the main, and if necessary, shorten the headsail,' he said. I glanced up at the feathery cirrus clouds, then looked into the cabin. The barometer had registered a significant drop. Signs of an oncoming gale. I turned *Galatea* into the wind to ease the main. Felix clipped his harness onto the jackline, crawled forward towards the mast, inserted the handle into the furling socket and started to reef the main. By the time he was back in the cockpit, gusts hit from ahead. Felix pulled in the main and I set the autopilot to keep us on course.

The moderate beam sea became increasingly confused as the waves from ahead built up. We felt *Galatea* toss unsteadily as the southerly wind and sea interrupted her passage. From the saloon came the clanking noises of the gimballed stove, the brass lamps, the plastic fruit bowl as it crashed against the steps, and instruments slid off the navigation table onto the floor.

By 7 pm, we had a howling gale, a dark sky and lumpy seas. Felix reefed the main further, shortened the headsail, but left the mizzen up to lessen the pitching and tossing. He put two washboards into the companionway to prevent waves flooding the cabin and left a small opening at the top. We still had a very long way to go. At best we'd reach Lipari in the early morning. Long before that, however, we would pass Stromboli.

I don't recall exactly at which point a spasm, an uncontrollable tremor, gripped my chin. I'd never experienced anything like it before. Then, an extraordinary sensation overwhelmed me and I relived the terror of being in the life raft during our 'Survival at Sea' test before we left Sydney. As the wind strength reached 35 to 40 knots, *Galatea* pitched and tossed, waves surfed across her deck. Aeoleus had opened the bag of winds with a godly vengeance. Felix put his arm around me and I clung to him. In spite of our lifelines, we tossed from side to side in the cockpit. Periodically, Felix went down to check our position on the radar.

'We'd better give the autohelm a rest,' he said.

'OK, I'll hand steer for a while.'

'Stromboli is on the radar. Twelve miles to go. There's also a ship 21 miles ahead, moving north-west, otherwise nothing.' We continued on in silence.

Then, out of the pre-dawn darkness, Stromboli, the volcano that has served as the oldest lighthouse in the world, appeared in all its majesty. Silhouetted against the sky and a full moon, it towered from the sea, and as we approached, it loomed immense. From its crown, bursts of fire erupted into the night sky at regular intervals, and rivers of glowing lava flowed down to the sea.

'Imagine how terrifying this must have been to ancient sailors, tossed in a gale, with this mountain of fire in the middle of the sea!'

'You don't have to be so ancient,' I mumbled, my jaw still in spasm.

As we crossed the moon's beam, I saw the dazzling whiteness of our deck, the waves' froth slipping back into the raging sea, the gleam of our shortened main and mizzen, and Felix's pale, strong face. From the saloon came the familiar clanking of the stove and brass lamps, and at one particular angle, a moonbeam shone through the narrow opening of the companionway into the saloon below — warm, dry and comforting.

And so *Galatea* battled on.

'Perhaps we should heave to,' Felix said, but then added, 'I think she's coping all right...' Instead of alternating watches, we stayed together on deck throughout the night, checking our position at regular intervals and monitoring the radar for vessels crossing our path.

After a night as long as eternity, imperceptible changes on the grey eastern horizon gave way to the pinks, reds and orange of the dawn. I watched the sun rise over the turbulent sea.

'Lipari's only 5 miles to go,' Felix announced.

The volcanic peaks of Lipari dipped vertically into the sea, gouged by quarrying and volcanic activity. Dust and wind partially blinded us as we approached the primitive wooden jetty. Wind bullets cascading from the hills caused chaos on the water, where eddying gusts chased one another.

'We'd better pull out and wait for a calm before we try to go alongside!' Felix shouted above the noise.

An hour later the *ormeggiatore* signalled us to come in to the only unoccupied space on the windward side of the jetty.

There was nothing available on the lee side. We hesitated at first, but then went alongside. We strung out all the fenders we had to dampen the thuds as we rose and fell. The water was boiling, the wind wild. The *ormeggiatore* took our lines.

'*Grazie.*'

'*Impossibile rimanere qui lungo tempo!* It's impossible to stay here long!'

'*Si, dove possiamo andare*, where can we go?'

He shrugged his shoulders and moved on. A woman whose boat was tied up on the lee side of the jetty came over. 'It's rough today, came out of nowhere last night. It was dead calm yesterday,' she said in a heavy Dutch accent. 'I think it'd be best if you moved to the other side of the bay.' She pointed to a spot crammed with boats tied up to each other.

She undid our lines and pushed out our bow. We made our way to Pignataro on the other side. It was packed with yachts trying to find shelter. Two boats moved to let us squeeze in between them and helped us tie up.

It was another long, rough, sleepless night.

The following morning the winds continued to blow mercilessly. Workmen came alongside the marina, which was in the process of being built.

'*Via, via…lavoro!*' We all had to move off.

'*Ach Gott,*' our German neighbour wailed, 'now we'll have to deal with the anchor mess.' This time the untangling of the spaghetti involved four boats.

'Doesn't look as if the wind is going to abate. We won't be able to go ashore.'

And so, one boat after another left Pignataro and battled into a southerly towards Milazzo in Sicily.

◎ ◎ ◎ ◎

chapter six

To be tied up along the quay in the centre of Milazzo, during the 1990 World Cup, when Italy was hosting the event, was an unforgettable experience. From dusk to dawn, cars and motorcycles roared up and down the esplanade, blaring horns. In the crowded trattorias and cafés along the harbour front, the mood mirrored the exploding fireworks. And above the pandemonium, Luciano Pavarotti's voice soared, '*VINCERA, VINCERA!*' The entire length of the marina was in celebration mood, toasting and singing. None of the yachties emerged on deck until late the next morning and instead of moving on, we stayed another three days to recover.

The Dutch couple on the boat next to us had come from Yugoslavia.

'It's such a tense place,' they said, 'we decided to spend the summer in Sicily instead. The political situation there is bad, the country seems to be falling apart.'

We'd heard how tense the situation was in Yugoslavia from a number of yachties. Most put it down to living for 40 years under communism and, now, its anticipated disintegration. Still, as we'd made arrangements to meet friends in Dubrovnik, we planned to move on.

Like Steve in Ischia, they also warned us about storms in the Golfo di Squillace, the waters south of Calabria. In case of a rough passage, they suggested we sail into a port that didn't appear on charts. In fact, theoretically, it didn't exist. 'But you can't miss the entrance. It's marked by a rusting, dilapidated yellow crane. The coordinates in case you need to go in there are Lat.38 19.54 N Long.16 26.04 E.'

We cast off from the quay at the crack of dawn. The purring of our engine broke the night's silence as we motored past moored container vessels, black silhouettes against a dark grey sky. A lone sailor stood on deck and waved. As we crossed the entrance lights to Milazzo's harbour and headed for the open sea, a streak of pink lined the sky, and soon the sun's arc appeared above the eastern horizon.

The wind, which had blown all night, now registered 25 knots dead on the nose. We set a course for Capo Rasocolmo and Capo Peloro, the most easterly tip of Sicily and the dogleg entrance to the Strait of Messina. On both sides of this entrance are steep mountains from which notorious squalls blow. Once we were inside the Strait, we sailed past modern swordfish-fishing vessels moving slowly up and down. This was swordfish season, and as we'd discovered in the markets, they fetched high prices.

In spring, swordfish migrate through the Strait in a southerly direction, but in June they travel north. They sleep or move very slowly during the day, which makes them easy targets for harpoons. Boats with massive steel lattice masts and a bowsprit longer than the length of the boat trawl for them. The captain steers from a perch in the crow's nest at the top of the mast, while men with binoculars scan the water. My stomach heaved as I watched them sway 90 degrees back and forth.

'Can you believe it?' I said looking at both sides of the Strait. 'We're passing the very spot where Odysseus met the monsters.'

On the mainland to port in Calabria lay the tiny harbour of Scilla. To starboard in Sicily was Charybdis. According to myth, sea monsters lay in wait on both sides of the narrow Strait — Scylla, with her twelve feet and six heads, waited in a cave on the eastern side of the Strait, ready to prey on dolphins, swordfish and sailors. On the western side was Charybdis, a raging whirlpool that could swallow whole ships.

In ancient times sailing through the Strait was perilous, yet some chose to risk this voyage rather than take the longer route around Sicily. Ships with powerful engines now have few problems negotiating these waters, but many yachts have had terrifying experiences. We stuck religiously to the Admiralty Pilot's advice to '…enter the northern end of the Strait at the beginning of a south-going stream which occurs four hours after high tide in Gibtaltar.' With the engine running, all sails drawing and a beam wind, we motored out of the Strait and entered Saline Ioniche in Calabria at 4 o'clock. We'd had a dream run.

'What sort of music would you like to celebrate rounding the toe of Italy?'

'*Canzoni Napoletani*, of course,' Felix replied.

Apart from a lone fishing vessel tied up to a long quay, Saline Ioniche, a newly built harbour with facilities for merchant ships, was empty. The two men on board the fishing boat waved and helped us tie up behind them.

In one corner of the port stood a square building several storeys high. It looked deserted. The silence was eerie. Late in the afternoon a French, a Dutch and two Norwegian yachts pulled in and dropped anchors in mid-harbour.

'I think we should have an early night and leave first thing in the morning.' Felix switched on the radio to get a forecast, but nothing came on air.

At 10 o'clock we heard a fishing boat tie up immediately behind us along the quay. Felix climbed out to see that all was OK, and mentioned that a few more yachts had pulled in, then got back into bed. I'd always admired his ability to wake up, do whatever he had to do, lie back and, within seconds, be fast asleep. Eventually I, too, got to sleep.

A sudden wild swaying and the thud of fenders shook us out of our bunks and sent us rushing onto the deck. 'Bloody boom's loose, watch your head!' Felix yelled. A howling wind whistled high-pitched tunes through the stays.

'It's registering 35!' I screamed back. Pandemonium reigned all around us. *Galatea*, the only yacht tied up to the quay, was sandwiched between two fishing vessels. Along the quay, fishermen were out in force, grappling with lines and fenders. Men shouted and engines roared, making ready to move off to the other side for shelter.

No matter how hard I turned the wheel, the force of waves crashing onto our deck pushed us back against the quay. Gesticulating and shouting instructions, two fishermen jumped on board to help us push *Galatea* out, as the stern of their boat threatened to climb onto our bow. We held our breath each time a wave heaved their stern aloft, then slipped and let it fall with a thud into the foaming water. At the same time, *Galatea* was rising and falling. Each time her bow heaved, my stomach sank.

'For Chrissake don't fend off with your leg!' Felix yelled. 'Go back to the wheel and turn as hard as you can!'

At the peak of one rise, the four of us succeeded in pushing our bow to port and extricating ourselves from the quay. I slumped with relief onto the cockpit seat. Felix took the wheel.

Silhouetted against the breakwater in mid-harbour, yachts swung perilously close to one another. Crews on deck shouted instructions into a ferocious wind. The Dutch boat's anchor had broken loose and its engine refused to start. Two of their men were in a dinghy. One grappled with the anchor chain while the other strained at the oars to hold their drifting boat off the French yacht. The French were on deck ready with fenders.

As we passed them, the Dutch yacht's engine came alive and they joined the procession of boats, a line of swaying masts and gleaming hulls, as they crossed the beam of a high moon towards shelter in the basin on the other side.

Although we were packed close to one another, we sensed the sighs of relief. Waves continued to crash onto the quay, but in our corner of the harbour it was comparatively quiet. Everyone had put down anchors, and helped to fend off or tie up drifting vessels. We felt warm and safe in our sheltered corner; the camaraderie was palpable, everyone kept watch and the night passed slowly. Most were too tired to talk.

But the dawn! The spectacular dawn that invariably follows a night when the wind has blown remorselessly. A plum red arc rose gradually from the sea and, as it lightened, apricot yellows chased the scarlets and, high above, fleecy cauliflower clouds scudded past. We took deep breaths. The long night was over.

We stood and gesticulated brief messages to people on other boats. The rough night was etched on our faces. Felix turned to me, 'Let's have breakfast, then you go down and get some sleep. I'll keep watch and sleep later.' It continued to blow all day. No matter how hard he tried, Felix couldn't get a forecast. Later, someone managed to get a Messina radio forecast for 'lessening winds' and passed on the message.

In the afternoon, we saw the two fishermen who'd helped us, mending nets on their deck. We called out, and asked them to come over. Looking pleased to have a break, they got into a dinghy and rowed across.

The older of the two was a short, stocky man, with a kind face, thick slate-grey hair, a network of wrinkles and spatulate hands. His shirt was shabby and buttoned at the neck, his trousers worn and turned up at the ankles. He looked in his 60s but was probably ten years younger. Fishing ages men quickly. Unlike his younger partner, he was shy and ill at ease as Felix took his line and helped him step on board. The younger man belonged to the cool, new generation, in the universal jeans, T-shirt and sneakers. Tall, muscular and bronzed, he exuded an air of confidence his companion lacked.

Inhibitions are shed more easily when you've shared a storm. Add a bottle of wine, and stories take off. The young man needed no prodding. With our Italian, his few words of English and some body language, we had no problems.

'This is a good harbour to be in when it blows a sirocco. To be outside in this *burasca* is no good. Before they built this harbour my father used to tell me, you were lucky not to drown. He was a fisherman too. But he's dead now. This is his brother, my uncle,' he said pointing to the older man. 'All the men in our family are fishermen. When we were growing up we wanted to learn something different, to have a better life. The government was going to bring industry to the South, but things didn't work out.

'Take this port. When they built it fifteen years ago, they made it big enough to handle ships up to 10 000 tonnes. They even built the rail tracks for transport. This factory over there...' he said, pointing to the large building at the corner of the port, 'it was going to employ 3000 people. We were going to can fruit and fish. But you know what, not a single person has ever worked in that factory. Nothing. The only people who use this port are fishermen or yachts looking for shelter. We're only allowed to come in if it's blowing, but we use it anyway even if we're not supposed to. The town is not too far away, but nobody comes here.' He was angry. The old man looked on, wistful. He listened but said nothing. Now and again he nodded.

'Why is that?' I asked.

'Why? Why? You ask?' His mouth curled in a sardonic smile, he looked at his uncle. They exchanged knowing looks and shrugged their shoulders. I saw in the gentle eyes of that older man the quintessential Southern Italian, who from birth had been taught to expect a life of hard work and subservience, to 'know his place'. He tilted his head to one side and smiled to himself.

After a short silence the young fisherman changed the subject.

'Australia is a good place? Easy to find work?'

'Yes, it's a good place. There are many Italians in Australia,' I said.

'I have a friend in Australia. He went there five years ago. He says it's very good there. I wanted to go when I got married but my wife didn't want to be away from her family. She said she'd rather I stayed a fisherman. I could go to the North, to Milano, Torino…plenty of work there, and good money. I could earn more there, but that's not so good for my wife. So I stayed here and I work with my uncle. This way at least I feel more free…'

When we'd emptied the bottle, they said they'd better get back to their nets.

Sometime later, the old man returned to give us two fish he'd gutted and cleaned for us.

'I wonder what the real story is about this place, this factory,' Felix said as we waved him goodbye.

'Not hard to work out,' I said. 'That building over there is a monument to bribery, greed, protection money and politics. When one reads about the millions spent trying to develop Italy's South, the *Mezzogiorno*, one can have a guess at how contracts were handed out, money syphoned off. Then someone didn't pay someone who should have paid someone else. So here's this huge complex that's never been used...they call it "*il problema del Mezzogiorno*".'

In the evening, a Dutchman and two Frenchmen came on board. As with the two fishermen, it was easy to establish a rapport. Trouble at sea breaks down most yachties' innate reserve. There's a shared experience you can talk about for hours, and invariably one story leads to another. Everyone has a story about a terrible passage. We all laughed, in that senseless way you laugh when you're very tired and you've had some wine. You don't need much on these occasions.

After two nights and a day the wind died down completely. When we stepped on deck in the morning, the boats were covered in sand and grit. 'Memento from North Africa.' The fishermen had warned us to expect that.

◎◎◎◎

'So we'll all leave very early tomorrow and meet in Roccella,' Stefan, one of the yachties said. 'Do you have the coordinates?' his mate André asked.

'Yes,' Felix pointed to the pencil mark on the chart. 'It's the only shelter between Saline and Crotone, a tiny harbour, never been completed. As you can see, not marked on any of the charts. The Dutch yachtie who told me about it said to look for a large abandoned yellow crane right near the entrance. But there are no lights, so you can't go in after dark.'

'OK, so we'll meet there tomorrow. Should get there in the afternoon. Better get some sleep now. Have a good sail everyone!'

We set off at 6. It was pleasant drifting in a light breeze along the Calabrian coast. The Aspromonte Massif, a steep mountain range, forms the tip of Calabria. Its many caves, gorges and densely wooded ravines are known as places where kidnappers hide victims. J. Paul Getty's grandson was abducted and hidden here in 1973, and it allegedly took a piece of his ear to convince the old man to pay the ransom. But none of this — the kidnappers, the Mafia, N'dragheta or Camorra — entered our minds as we sailed on this summer's day.

By 11, however, the wind had died down, the sea was glassy and the headsail hung limp. The sun beat through the haze and our faces were bright red.

'It'll take forever to get there at this rate. I'll take down the main and the headsail, and we should start the engine.' I waited while Felix took down the sails, then turned the ignition key. The engine revved and I put her into gear.

CLONCK!

'SHIT!...Something's collapsed.'

Felix leapt into the cockpit, took the wheel and tried to shift the gear handle.

CLONCK!

'Doesn't sound good.' He stepped down the gangway and removed the partitions around the engine. I stayed on deck. It was dead calm and we were drifting with the slight movement of the sea. The other yachts, all under motor, had now passed us and were too far away to see that we were in trouble. Steve's warning rang in my ears. '...an absolute lull can mean a blow on the way. This place wasn't called the Gulf of Squalls for nothing. It terrified old mariners hundreds of years ago. It still does...'

Before leaving Saline we'd agreed to stay in radio contact with André on channel 16. 'Call the *Mistique*! Tell them we have no engine, so they'll know what happened in case we don't make it to Roccella.' I turned on the VHF and called them several times, but there was no reply.

'They must have forgotten to turn on the radio.'

'I have this terrible feeling it's the gearbox, probably a broken drive plate,' Felix said.

My stomach sank.

'We'll have to put up the sails again and hope we get some wind. It's still a long way to Roccella. And we can't go in after dark.'

The sails hung limp, the air smelt hot and gritty, the cockpit was like an oven. I took a bucket, scooped sea water and tossed it on the deck. I felt my head pound.

Felix handed me a wet tea towel. 'Here honey, put this on your head.'

'What'll we do?' I was talking to myself.

'We can always pray.'

'Don't be funny, I can't take it.'

Felix looked up at the sails, then shook his head. He went down to the VHF and tried several times to raise one of the yachts, but there was no response. At 2 o'clock, scattered clouds hid the sun. Then a sudden breeze swung the boom to port, the mainsail flapped, and we started to move. Felix gave me a hug, and I burst out laughing. The breeze steadied and we made good progress.

At 7, the large yellow crane appeared, and we made straight for it. An hour and a half later we were at the entrance to Roccella. All the yachts were at anchor in crystal water, and everyone was on deck in a riotous mood, nursing drinks.

'Let's hope our anchor grips,' Felix looked worn out. 'Without an engine, it'll be heavy work to pick it up and try again.' But we were in luck. It gripped first go.

'We tried to call when we lost sight of you, but you didn't answer. What happened to you?' André asked.

'We tried to call you too, but didn't get any response. We've got a major problem, I think it's the gearbox. We'll have to try and get a mechanic.'

As suggestions started to fly, a speedboat of the coastal patrol, the Guardia di Finanza, approached. '*Via!* Prohibited to stay here, this is not a port! Nobody is permitted to stay here!'

'But why not?' everyone pleaded. 'The next place is Crotone. Why can't we stay, just till tomorrow morning?'

Felix and I didn't move. We said nothing. As the others reluctantly pulled up anchors and we didn't, the Guardia came alongside.

'We have a major breakdown...*no motore, motore non funziona...*' But they were not convinced. The three officers went into a huddle, then one climbed on board.

Felix turned on the ignition and tried to put her into gear. CLONCK!

'We'll need a mechanic, *un meccanico*?' They looked at each other.

'*Non so*, don't know.' *Il capitano* shook his head. 'OK, you can stay for one night only, *soltanto una notte*.' My heart sank.

We watched the yachts motor past the yellow crane and head east towards Crotone. The Guardia di Finanza also left. It was after 9, and soon it would be dark. Scattered stars and a pencil outline of the moon appeared over the range. On the peak of a distant hill stood the ruin of an ancient castle. We were alone, and the silence was uncanny.

'What do we do now?' The monotonous lapping of water rolling on shore made me nervous. Felix sensed my apprehension. 'It's morning in Sydney, a good time to radio Ken. I won't waste time trying a station here, I'll go through Berne Radio.'

Ken Evans, our Sydney mechanic with the magic touch who could fix anything, find the most elusive of spare parts and remember the structure and idiosyncrasies of every boat engine he touched, answered the phone.

'Hi Ken, Felix here.'

'G'day Felix, where the hell are ya?'

'In Calabria, middle of nowhere, bottom of Italy. Listen, Ken, I've got a broken drive plate, I think. What do'ya reckon, any good ideas?'

'Jeesus, Felix, you're in deep shit mate.'

'Thought so, Ken. What d'ya reckon?'

'You'll have to get a new one. As I recall, you've got a Nissan truck engine, so you'll have to lift out the whole bloody engine to get to it. Are ya close to a decent diesel mechanic?'

'Ya kidding? I'm in the middle of the wilderness...and they don't use Nissan engines here. God knows how I'd get a spare...'

'If ya get a decent mechanic he should be able to adapt one...if ya can't, I might even cannibalise an old engine I've got here in me backyard. You're sure in a mess, mate...don't know what else I can suggest...Let me know how ya get on. Yeah, deep shit all right!'

'Thanks Ken...I'll let ya know...'

'OK, good luck, mate.'

We continued to sit in the cockpit. The moon was high now, hanging like a lantern in a translucent sky. The shore was an opaque black, the water around us rippled diamonds and *Galatea* rocked gently. I was homesick and frightened.

'I guess we'd better hit the bunk, try to sleep and wait till morning. Don't worry, honey, it'll be OK.' Felix put his arm around me.

In the morning two fishermen's boats were tied up to a small wooden pontoon. Felix rowed across and asked them about a mechanic. They didn't know one. But he did find out that the word for a drive plate in Italian is *parastrappe.*

Somewhere in our travels, we'd picked up an Italian handbook called *Pagine Azzurre*, a yearly publication with useful information and charts of every harbour in Italy, which included phone numbers for mechanics and repair shops. Although nothing was listed for Roccella Ionica, we did find the name of a diesel mechanic in Crotone, about 110 km away. Berne Radio connected us with him.

Felix strung words together and explained our problem to Signor Tisso, who agreed to come at 9 the following morning to confirm the provisional diagnosis. For the rest of the day we sat in the cockpit, and watched the fishermen do odd jobs on their boats. Late in the evening, the Guardia di Finanza chased out all the yachts that had come in during the day, and then paid us a visit. We explained that a mechanic from Crotone was coming the following morning.

'OK, you can stay, *soltanto una notte*! One night only!'

Another silent, lonely night followed.

At 9 o'clock the next morning, Signor Tisso and his two apprentices waved to us from the pontoon. He was a small stocky man, with dark eyes and an earnest face, immaculate in white trousers and shirt. His two young assistants, their hair groomed and glazed, wore ironed jeans and spotless white

T-shirts. They held a pile of cardboard sheets under their arms, which they spread on the floor as soon as they stepped on board. They'd also brought a bundle of neatly folded, white laundered rags, the remains of torn sheets.

Signor Tisso used words sparingly, and supervised his minions *sotto voce* as they followed his instructions. When enough had been dismantled, he bent down to inspect. He tested the starter motor, put the gear handle into forward and heard the CLONCK.

'The *parastrappa è rota*, the drive plate is broken. We will need to take the gearbox off the engine, then I must find one that will be the right size. There are no Nissan diesel engines here. It is *un grande problema*...I shall come back *domani*, tomorrow.'

As he was telling us about the *grande problema*, the Guardia di Finanza came on board. Tisso talked to them at length, confirmed that we couldn't use our engine, and as the forecast was for another sirocco, added that it would be irresponsible for them to force us to move. They were clearly displeased.

Each morning, Tisso and his assistants drove for three hours each way along the mountain roads and arrived between 8 and 9, spotlessly attired. On the third day I mentioned that I planned to walk to the nearest village to buy bread.

'No, no, no, *è impossibile* to have a woman walk by herself.' Tisso was aghast.

'Why not?'

'No, no...*è impossibile*,' he repeated.

'Then I will send *mio marito*, my husband.'

'No, no, no, you cannot stay alone on a boat...I will bring you bread every day...'

'But we're also running out of fresh food.'

'I will drive you to a shop at lunchtime.'

At 1 o'clock we set off in his station wagon. The road, dusty and uneven, ran between the sea on one side and a rocky hillside on the other. The air was hot and dry and smelt of salt.

I wondered why he was so emphatic about not letting me walk alone, but I hesitated to ask. He was a taciturn man who didn't invite conversation. In any case, I concluded, ignoring his advice would be unwise. I was a woman, and this was the South. Tisso stopped in front of the first shop. A middle-aged, barrel-bellied man with a furrowed face stood perusing the street, his hands behind his back. Boxes of tomatoes, cucumbers, zucchini, stone fruit, grapes, artichokes, eggplant and onions lined the footpath, exuding a mixture of summer fragrance and the smell of over-ripe fruit and vegetables.

Dressed in a checked shirt, worn trousers and dusty shoes, the man greeted us with a puzzled smile. '*Prego?*'

Tisso introduced me as *una inglese*.

'Ah, you are English?' the man asked in English.

'No, Australian,' I replied.

'Where in Australia?'

'Sydney.'

'Sydney?' His face exploded into a network of smiles. 'We lived in Sydney for many years!'

'Where?'

'In Leichhardt, Five Dock, Ashfield.'

'When did you come back?'

'Twelve years ago.' Then, turning towards the shop, he shouted, 'Maria, Maria, *vieni*! Come here, *una signora di* Sydney!'

Maria, a plump woman with a large navy apron tied around her waist, rushed out.

'*Ah signora, di* Sydney?' she was incredulous.

'*Signora*, what can I get you?' the man beamed with excitement.

'I'd like fruit and cheeses...I've run out of most things. We're stuck in the harbour with engine trouble, and Signor Tisso here is helping us.' I pointed to salamis and cheeses behind the counter, and fruit and vegetables out the front.

'Maria, not these! Bring the fresh stuff from the back!' He snapped in Italian. Tisso looked on in amazement as the couple rushed to the back of the shop and brought out fresh salamis, cheeses, eggs, fruit...

The shopping took longer than he'd expected, and when Maria offered us coffee he declined, '...*Mi dispiace, abbiamo fretta*, so sorry, we're in a hurry.'

After I'd paid, Maria handed me a small parcel of biscuits. 'I baked these this morning, please take them,' and as she shook my hand, added, 'I want to feel a little piece of Sydney, we miss Sydney so much!'

We piled everything into the car. '*Grazie, ciao!*' I waved.

On the way back Signor Tisso didn't utter a word. But each day he brought us fresh bread. From his workshop in Crotone, Tisso phoned Milan, Turin, Genoa, Naples, Bari and Taranto in search of a drive plate that he could modify. After five days, even he looked distressed. The Guardia di Finanza continued to come on board each day to check our progress.

◎ ◎ ◎ ◎

It was our sixth night. I couldn't sleep. A sliver of moon peeped over the rugged Calabrian mountain range, a black silhouette against a navy sky. I was restless and frightened. Alone in the cockpit, I looked around this tiny unmarked harbour. Why did the police chase everyone out every evening? Why did they come on board to check on us every day? By 3 o'clock, the moon had set, and the only sound was the obsessive rhythm of waves rolling back and forth on the sandy shore. In Australia, this lonely bay would have seemed enchanted, but here it felt haunted.

The quiet purring of an approaching engine broke the silence. Turning towards it, I saw the dark outline of a small fishing boat. Its shape looked familiar. As it neared the pier, a man jumped ashore to tie up the vessel. Must be the fishermen back, I thought. The ones we'd met on the first day who told us that *parastrappe* is the Italian word for drive plate. A truly useful bit of vocabulary. At least we won't be alone now. I watched them come in, but I was too depressed to wave or call out '*Ciao!*' I just sat and watched them tie up.

Why were they so quiet? Why this strange silence? Suddenly fear gripped me. Something urged me to shift from the centre of the cockpit where they could see me silhouetted against the night sky. I moved and pressed my body against the side of the coach house.

Then, through the darkness, car headlights, like two reversed sword blades, pierced the windows of the fishermen's coach house onto the water. They pulled up next to the fishing boat, the lights were switched off, and I saw the outline of a limousine.

A soundless transaction took place. My heart raced, I wanted to slip into the saloon but was riveted to the seat. I heard a car door close, saw headlights turned on, the car drive off. As soon as it was out of sight, all was silent again. Seconds later, another set of headlights approached. The car pulled up. A transaction. Silence.

Terror unlocked me from my seat. I dived downstairs, rushed to the aft cabin and shook Felix.

'What's the problem?'

'Wake up! Quickly! Do you know where we are?'

'We're in Calabria. For God's sake, go to sleep!'

'No, no, this isn't me being disoriented. Quick, have a look out of the porthole. I know now why they're chasing people out...something's going on here...we mustn't be seen...'

He shot out of bed just as the second car left. Minutes later the fishermen turned on their engine and pulled away, making for the exit, out to sea.

'What d'you reckon?'

'Drugs.'

'That's why they chase all the boats out. We're in Mafia territory.'

We sat up the rest of the night. Tisso had said there was some hope of finding a drive plate in Taranto. He would send one of the boys there. He'd let us know in the morning. But the following morning he didn't turn up.

We were the only boat in the harbour and all around us there was frantic commotion. The Guardia di Finanza had closed the entrance to stop anyone entering the port. Police cars and armoured cars with loudspeakers patrolled on shore. A helicopter hovered low over us. A naval patrol boat with guns entered the harbour. We ducked downstairs for cover and didn't dare look out of the portholes.

'This is a mad movie.'

'Not a movie. It's for real!'

It was over in less than an hour.

'Must have been a raid the authorities have been preparing for.'

At 3 o'clock, Signor Tisso turned up. He'd left home as usual at 5.30 in the morning to cover the 110 km over winding roads to get to us, but all the roads had been blocked off. He must have known what the commotion was about. Everyone in the area must have known. One couldn't live in Calabria and not know. We were the only ones who didn't suspect what was going on here.

But Tisso brought us good news. He'd located two drive plates — one in Taranto, another in Genoa. He'd sent one of the boys to Taranto to pick up the one that he could modify to fit. He would also get the second one, modify it and give it to us as a spare when we got to Crotone. It would take another two or three days of work.

'We'd better get hold of all the people we'd arranged to meet, tell them we won't be able to make it...maybe Susie and Simon can meet us in Crotone instead of Otranto. Then there's Diana and Sol we're supposed to meet in Dubrovnik.'

Tisso continued to supervise the boys, and they followed his instructions. They worked for two long tense days to ensure we left as soon as possible. When they had finished, we took *Galatea* on a trial run. Tisso and Felix looked pleased. But the tension had exhausted me. Susie and Simon arrived by taxi from Reggio Calabria on the afternoon of our last day and marvelled at the idyllic location. They suggested we stay. But I couldn't get away fast enough.

The following morning we set sail for Crotone where we met Tisso and paid him. For eight days, he had travelled three hours each way. As Ken Evans had forecast, and as Felix knew, it was a big job, and an expensive one. And yet Tisso's bill was exactly what Felix had calculated it would have cost in Australia. He could have charged anything he wanted, and we would have paid without a murmur, but he didn't.

In parting, he told us that had we arrived in Crotone with that same problem, it would have taken at least four weeks before he would have started on the job. The reason he gave for travelling the 110 km each way for eight days was that he'd been so worried about us, alone in that spot. At no stage did the words 'Mafia' or 'N'dragheta' or 'Camorra' cross his lips.

Hi Kids,

What a relief to talk to you from Otranto. I sometimes wondered whether we'd ever get away from Roccella. I think the place will always be our most memorable port, let alone experience.

The Adriatic behaved impeccably during our crossing to Yugoslavia. We stopped midway, had a swim, drank to 'THIS IS US CROSSING THE ADRIATIC!' and watched a golden sunset.

Dubrovnik is beautiful, the quintessential Mediterranean picture postcard. Port formalities required *three* people to come on board. One to ensure we had no guns, one to stamp passports and another to write a list of people on board. That's one way to solve unemployment. The mail here is erratic, so a yachtie returning home tomorrow has volunteered to post this in Austria. Shall write a long letter soon.

Love, from Us Two

At the end of that summer, Italian friends told us they'd read that one couple had been shot on the beach at Roccella Ionica because 'they'd seen what they shouldn't have'. Also, a young boy had been killed there because he'd 'talked'.

chapter seven

For centuries the Adriatic had been a Venetian lake, a long corridor that connected seaboard towns and villages to Venice, the heart of the Venetian Empire. It is close to 650 km as the crow flies from Albania to Istria at the northern tip of the Adriatic, 3220 km if one follows the islands, bays and inlets.

Harbours, lighthouses, churches, bell towers, piazzas and the ubiquitous winged lion of St Mark all allude to the reach of Venetian power and influence, which attained its apogee in the fifteenth century. It was a time when navigators hugged the shoreline, and trading posts were rarely more than one day's sailing apart.

The beauty and proximity of coastal towns, villages and islands attract today's yachtsmen to the Dalmatian coast. And we, like the sailors and merchants of old, planned to move from place to place, stroll ashore, eat and drink, watch the passing parade, and explore the sights.

When we arrived in Dubrovnik, we sensed uneasiness in the air. Ethnic tensions were about to erupt into conflict, and the years of Yugoslav communism were coming to an end. It took us a few days to understand how the prevailing command economy functioned.

When I broke our broomstick, Felix said, 'Don't worry, we'll buy another one ashore.' But the bear-like man in the hardware store smiled and shook his head. 'We had broomsticks last winter,' he explained in an amalgam of Italian, German and Serbo-Croat, 'but we didn't have the brushes. Now we have the brushes. Maybe we will have the sticks in a few weeks. Maybe next year. If people want a broom,' he continued to enlighten us, 'they buy whatever is available and hope to pick up the rest some other time.' We thanked him and moved on, clutching our shopping list for globes, diesel oil, a rubber belt, bolts…

The elderly man with a heavy black moustache looked puzzled. 'Diesel oil?' he repeated, 'but we always use ordinary oil, we don't keep diesel oil.' Undeterred, Felix continued down the list. The fellow shook his head and looked sadder with each item. But as we were about to leave, he beamed when a thought suddenly occurred to him: 'We've just got in some WD-40.'

'Thanks, we have plenty of WD-40.' Now Felix shook his head and looked sad.

Loud music added to the frenetic atmosphere on the marina. Attendants were busy with yachts and tourists, but the mood was different from Italy and France.

'There is little *joie de vivre* here,' Felix commented to our neighbour on the Austrian boat. '*Joie de vivre?*' she replied. 'Not among the locals. They're pretty cranky.'

We were sipping coffee. Suddenly Felix jumped ashore and ran after a young man, shouting, 'What the hell do you think you're doing!' He made to grab the fellow, who shot off. I'd never seen Felix so angry. 'The bastard pulled our plug out of the power point and threw it into the water!'

'Who is he?'

'A marina attendant.'

'Why would he do that?'

'No idea.'

'I guess that's what the yachties in Sicily had warned us about.'

The Germans on our other side saw the performance and shook their heads.

'They're more tense than usual this year. We've been coming here year after year, and it's never been like this…come over, have a drink.'

'Thank you, I need one after that. But I'll have to dry the plug first or connect another one.'

'It's strange,' I said, as we stepped into their cockpit, 'in France and Italy most attendants look happy. Here, everyone looks so angry.'

'The political situation is bad — hard to get jobs, inflation. Visitors complain because they can't get what they want, but the locals need tourism to boost their economy. It's frustrating for everyone.'

Two women lugging bags of fruit and vegetables stepped on board. 'Where did you get all this?' I asked. 'When I went into the supermarket it was empty. All I saw was a dozen eggs on one shelf, wilted vegetables on another, and a few tins.'

'Oh, we've learnt to shop when the farmers come to town and set up stalls. That's the only way to find anything fresh. We bring tins and non-perishable food from home. As for meat, you buy what you can get before 11. By 11.30 it's all gone.'

'This morning, I saw meat suspended on hooks or on blocks of wood with no ice in this temperature. The butcher was hacking away with an axe!' I said.

Walter and Inge were lawyers from Cologne. They kept their boat in Dubrovnik and spent summer vacations along the Dalmatian coast. From them, we learnt where to find fresh fruit and vegetables, which restaurants served reasonable food, and which bays and inlets were good for shelter.

But Yugoslavia was not Walter and Inge's main concern. They returned time and again to the problems of East Germany and the consequences of the fall of the Berlin Wall.

'It's all exciting, but we expect huge problems, psychological and economic. We're well off in West Germany. The East Germans resent the conditions under which they lived, and are likely to continue to live for a long time. They're so far behind us. We'll have to get used to their resentment, it's inevitable.'

Inge and Walter sailed south the following day, and we continued north into a bay on the island of Mljet, where the sky glowed at night, and gypsy music drifted in from the shore. We found Korcula the most interesting of the islands, perhaps because it had so many traces of its golden age when it was part of the Venetian Empire. We tied up at the marina, not far from where Venetian galleys once rode at anchor and Christianity faced Ottoman Islam.

In Split, on the mainland, we made the mistake of walking into a restaurant in Diocletian's Palace one evening. It was eerily dark and, apart from five men heavily into vodka at one table, the place was empty. It was the first time we'd felt unsafe. They were angry, thumping the table as they watched Milosovic address a crowd on television. Sensing that something serious was brewing, we kept our eyes well down on our plates, ate as fast as we could and fled Split the following morning. We decided the islands were more to our liking.

When we rowed ashore in a bay outside Rab late one afternoon, we noticed a young man sitting on a rock. He was stooped, gazing into the distance. His fair hair hung over one side of his forehead, and his face looked gentle. I thought he was fishing until I noticed him suck hard on a cigarette.

'Strange to be so tense in such a peaceful setting,' Felix said as we rowed past him. We tied up to a tree and walked along the beach towards him.

The young man turned, gave us a melancholy smile, and said, 'Are you from that Australian boat?'

'Yes.'

His English was hesitant. 'We had an Australian boat staying on the marina for the whole winter last year.'

'Actually, we intended to leave our boat in Umag this winter, but we've decided to leave it in Italy, in Lignano instead.'

'I don't blame you.'

'Why do you say that? Do you mind if we join you?'

'Please,' he motioned for us to sit. 'Anyone can see what's going to happen.' Then, as if speaking to himself, he added, 'I'd leave too if I could.'

'Are you from here? From Rab?'

'No, I work here. Only for the summer. I'm from Zagreb. At university. I'm a history student.'

'So you'll go back at the end of the holidays.'

He gave an ironic chuckle, 'God only knows. I was born in Zagreb. I grew up there. My mother is Croat. My father was Bosnian. Moslem. He died two years ago. We were Yugoslavs, didn't worry about religion. My grandfather fought with Tito. Tito kept us together. In the city we didn't care where people came from. We were all mixed, all Yugoslavs. Now things will fall apart. Nationalism. Serbs against Croats, Muslims against Christians. Milosovic wants a Greater Serbia, to avenge a battle they lost 600 years ago!'

Overwhelmed with emotion, he kept talking to himself as much as to us. 'In the old countries in Europe it doesn't take much to whip up hatreds. I know all about it. I study history.' He sucked on the remains of his cigarette butt, tossed it into the water, then lit another. 'I don't know why I'm telling you all this. I suppose because you are strangers, and I can practise my English,' he laughed. 'You know, one has to be careful who one talks to here.' He was silent for a while, then stopped musing and changed the subject.

'Umag is a good marina, but you're right not to leave the boat along the Yugoslav coast, it won't be safe.'

'When we were in Split,' Felix started, 'we noticed a lot of tension in the air. People seemed depressed and angry.'

'Yes, we are depressed and angry and poor. But we have our pride. We see tourists. They are wealthy, have a good life. Sometimes they treat us badly. But we need them, and we're jealous. Our money is worthless. Yes, we're worried and tense. We have no jobs, except summer tourism. Yugoslavia is breaking up, each ethnic group is against the other. When the Berlin Wall collapsed, East Germans were freed. They can now go to West Germany. They moved from communism to democracy. With us, it's different. We are moving from communism to nationalism.

'I would like to go to a new country. Like America or Australia or Canada. These are places where you can get away from the ethnic problems we have here. But we can't go anywhere, can't get visas. And we'll have war, fight each other.'

He dragged long and hard on his cigarette. Then, as if aroused from a restless sleep, he shook his head and got up abruptly. 'Yes, this is a beautiful country...for tourists.' And with that he threw his cigarette into the water, and walked away.

Dear Kids,
The coastline, the islands, inlets and bays in Yugoslavia are a sailor's paradise.

In Dubrovnik we walked into a street off the main drag and saw an old synagogue which dates back to the time of the Spanish Inquisition, when Jews sought a haven here. They were restricted to one street, until they were liberated by Napoleon. Of the 75 000 Jews in Yugoslavia before World War II, some 60 000 were killed. A cousin of my mother, her husband and two teenage boys lived in a place called Murska Sobota. I stayed with them for a week in 1937. The husband and boys were shot, and she jumped off the train that was transporting her to…?

Life for the locals is so tough that as tourists we feel ill at ease, even guilty. So much so, we'll be glad to get to Italy.

We're suffering from travel indigestion, but a few days in a quiet bay and we're eager to go on. Dad's main problem is that when he's tired, he tends to lose his balance. I have a new problem. When I bump against anything hard or sharp, flaps of skin flake off my forearm (the result of all the steroid ointment I've been using for my rashes). Dad has become an expert plastic surgeon, doing skin grafts on the run. Fortunately, we came well equipped from Italy. I'm learning not to throw my arms around, which is very difficult. How else can I communicate?

As we move closer to Trieste, I am more apprehensive. Memories of 60 years ago. I have started dreaming about that lifetime away. When we get to Trieste we plan to pick up the car from Florence, park it next to *Galatea*, and spend a leisurely 'remembrance of things past'. I'm angst-ridden and curious.

Hope you're all well,

Lots of love from the roving gypsies

For me, sailing north towards Trieste at the northern tip of the Adriatic evoked a more complex emotion from that of the ordinary yachties' delight in cruising the Adriatic coast. It rekindled childhood memories that had lain dormant for decades. After my mother's death, I was sent to live in Trieste with distant relatives I'd only met once in my life. Felix felt my apprehension. I didn't need to tell him.

My heart beat faster as an offshore breeze fluttered our sails and we drifted north along the Istrian coast. The only sounds were of people calling out on the shore and the sea slapping against our hull. Bright beach umbrellas and deckchairs dotted the coastline. Crowds lazed on the sand. I tasted a familiar scent of high summer as tears rolled down my cheeks and my finger traced place names on our map — Pula, Rovinj, Piran, Koper, Opatija, Rijeka. But the names that rang in my ears were Italian — Pola, Rovigno, Pirano, Capodistria, Abbazia, Fiume. How long was it since I'd learnt to swim in these waters, holidayed in Abbazia, crossed the bridge at Fiume into Yugoslavia to visit friends in Susak? Almost 55 years?

Intense nostalgia, not homesickness, overwhelmed me as we neared Trieste. I felt the apprehension that had gripped me the first time I approached this coast in 1936. I recalled standing on tiptoes and levering myself onto the ship's handrails to get my first glimpse of Trieste and the turrets of Miramare, a fairytale castle on the promontory. I watched the ship near the quay, where an excited crowd stood and waved.

As I looked up at *Galatea*'s billowing sails, the pain of long ago welled inside me. I recalled my father's hand holding mine as we climbed the ship's gangplank in Haifa harbour. I heard sounds of excitement, and smelt the ship's paint.

It was eight days after my mother's funeral, and I assumed my father had taken me to see a big ship and farewell the distant aunt whom I'd met only once. 'You have to call her "Tante",' he told me. But nobody had told me that I'd be leaving Haifa. Or that I might never see my family, my friends or my home again. That I would now live in Italy.

As my father and Tante chatted, I moved away to watch children play deck quoits. I took no notice when my father gave me a hug and a kiss. I was more interested in the children's games. Minutes later, I noticed the ship move from the wharf. Wild panic gripped me. I looked frantically for my father but he was gone. In a mad frenzy I screamed, '*Aba! Aba!* Dad! Dad! Don't leave me! Don't leave me!'

Tante gripped my hand, 'Let's go down to the cabin,' she said in German.

'I don't want to! I don't want to!' I shouted in Hebrew as I threw myself onto the deck, thrashing my arms and legs in a frenzy.

Two sailors tackled me and lifted me off the deck. Like a trapped animal, I clung to handrails leading down to the cabins. One grabbed me around the waist while the other struggled to prize open my grip on the rails. As he loosened one finger, I clamped down another. I kicked as they dragged me down, step by step. All around, men, women and children watched me battle the sailors. They dragged me howling along the corridor and thrust me onto a top bunk. Tante followed them and climbed the ladder to reach me. I pushed her. She fell back onto the floor. I erupted into uncontrollable laughter.

'You're a wild animal!' she screamed.

For the duration of the five-day voyage, the only words I said were '*Ani lo rotza!* I don't want to!' I refused to go to the dining room. Much of the time I was nauseated.

But each morning and afternoon, when trolleys appeared laden with cakes, biscuits and drinks, I stuffed myself until I vomited. I'd never seen cakes smothered in chocolate and whipped cream before. People stared. I didn't speak to anyone. No one spoke to me. The ship stopped twice, in Cyprus and in Bari, but we stayed on board.

By the time we reached Trieste, five days later, I was exhausted and tamed. As our ship, the *Galileo*, tied up to the quay, I saw in the crowd on shore a man who was a head taller than anyone, waving a white handkerchief.

'Look, that's Onkel!' Tante said pointing to him.

'He's as tall as a giraffe,' I thought, and craned my neck to see his face. Noise, commotion and the pungent smell of people packed against the rails made me feel sick. Seconds after the gangway was lowered, I tried to race down and escape. But Tante caught me and dragged me back. She held my wrist so tight I thought she'd broken it. My heart pounded as she dragged me kicking to Onkel. His face beamed kindness but I didn't let him touch me. I didn't want anyone to touch me. Onkel, I learnt years later, was a cousin of my grandmother.

Tante and Onkel spoke German. Although I didn't speak it, I gathered Tante was telling him what a terrible time she'd had with me. I was glad. I wanted to punish her for taking me.

A man collected our suitcases. I thought he belonged to their family, but was later told that he was the 'chauffeur'. I didn't know what that meant. I looked out of the car window as we drove to my new home. My head spun, I was carsick. They stopped, let me out, told me to take deep breaths, and waited.

A tram came towards us. I'd never seen one before. It wasn't like a bus or a cart and donkey I was used to. The houses we passed were larger and more ornate than any I'd ever seen. They weren't white. They were painted in pastel shades of ochre, yellow and pink. I looked for Arabs but saw none. No donkeys either. The policemen didn't look like British police. Flags flew on the top of buildings. Red, white and green with a square pattern in the middle.

'Here we are!' Tante said as we approached a large green metal gate and a high brick wall covered in creepers and white flowers. As I stepped out of the car, a sweet scent enfolded me. Onkel rang a bell, the gate buzzed open and I saw a three-storey house.

'*Buongiorno, signora, buongiorno*, Rina!' A young woman with a friendly face and curly brown hair, in a black dress and white apron, came to meet us. How did she know my name? Who was she?

'*Buongiorno*, Berta,' Tante replied. Berta gave me a brief hug before I could stop her. I let her hold my hand and we entered a hushed garden. I'd never seen a garden like this before. A large, round stone table stood in one corner under a pergola covered in leaves and green fruit. Flowerbeds in jigsaw patterns and bright colours filled the side garden. A tiny bird with a black head and red chest skipped from branch to branch in a fruit tree. A yellow butterfly fluttered past my face.

Berta's hand was soft and gentle. She chatted in Italian, and must have thought I'd understand. I looked to the left and right as we passed through a large entrance hall, past rooms with ornate furniture, chandeliers and cabinets with porcelain figurines. Berta led me upstairs into a smaller room, put down my case and said, '*Questa è tua stanza*.' Maybe this meant that this was where I'd sleep. There was a big divan, a large desk and chair, and a tall cupboard with glass cabinets on either side. They were empty. I was puzzled. I'd never had a room of my own or a cupboard to myself, or even slept alone in a room. I walked over to the window and looked down. A huge tree reached my window and shaded the side garden.

'*Vieni*,' Berta said, and taking my hand once more, she led me downstairs to the kitchen. A large white bowl with the remains of melted chocolate stood on the table. She stuck a finger into it, licked it, then passed it to me. I took the bowl and licked the rest. Dear Berta knew better than anyone how to handle me. Whenever I was in trouble, I ran to her for consolation. When we left Trieste almost three years later, I knew I'd never see her again.

◎ ◎ ◎ ◎

Fifty-five years later, as *Galatea* drifted closer to the Trieste Yacht Club marina, my heartbeat quickened and my throat was dry. My memory of that first night many years ago was so vivid — how I folded my clothes onto a chair, then stood it against the open door to make sure I had light from the corridor, and heard the sound of voices from downstairs. I remembered crawling into bed and feeling its softness, so different from the narrow bed I'd been used to, and how I lay on my back, and followed the beams of the lighthouse as they crossed my face at regular intervals. Then fear gripped me. Fear that I'd forget my home. I remembered praying for the first time, and realising that I knew no prayers, but hoped God would still listen to me and make sure I didn't forget the people I loved. Like an incantation, I recited their names, starting with my mother and father and brother and grandmother and my aunts and my friends — Rutti, Carmela,

Nechama, Yael, Sarale, Miriam…When I'd exhausted the list, I pulled the sheet over my face and cried myself to sleep. And that was the ritual I followed every night.

◎◎◎◎

It was the end of the school year when Tante and I arrived in Trieste, so for the following three months tutors came each day to prepare me for the school entrance exams in September. First, I had to learn the Latin alphabet, then to read, write and speak Italian as well as study Italian history, geography and maths, not to mention the glory of Fascism and love for the Duce. Years later, I learnt how this had upset the family but they didn't know what to do about it. For good measure, a Hebrew teacher came twice a week to ensure that I retained my mother tongue. I liked all my tutors and enjoyed the lessons.

But I was terrified of Tante's mother, Grossmutter Rosa. For Grossmutter Rosa I was the wildest, most ill-mannered child she had ever met. Her mission was to tame me, teach me good manners, to curtsey, and of course, to speak German. I dreaded the evenings after dinner when she brought out grammar books and *Grimms Fairy Tales*, which added to my nightmares.

As I had no one to play with, I drifted towards the unused part of the back garden, where three citrus trees grew and scent wafted among overgrown shrubs and bushes. Here, I built my cubby house. I loved to sit on the pile of leaves I'd collected, and be transported into another world. Sometimes I heard my father play his violin, or my mother sing her favourite plaintive song about dreaming. My mother's voice, or the sound of my father's violin, made me cry. Occasionally, when puffs of breeze made the leaves shiver and sun rays sketched patterns on the ground, I'd see shadows dance and become spirits in the world I'd created in my cubby. Then I'd get up and start to dance with them. And as I danced, I prayed that they would turn me into a spirit, so that I could join their world. Now and again I saw tombstones slip forward slowly, followed by an upward sweep of shroud-like streaks rising from graves. When that happened, I'd rush into the open front garden, panic-stricken with fear, too terrified to wait and see what would happen next.

The best friend I had was Berta. The first time I went shopping with her, we passed a troupe of uniformed school-children marching with their arms up in a straight salute. At the head of the file were boys holding raised flags and beating drums. I was mesmerised. 'What's this?' I asked.

'*Balilla, piccole italiane, fascisti.* It's the last day of school,' she said as she dragged me away. As soon as we were home, I rushed to Tante. 'Can I go to this school with the uniforms and the flags and everything?'

'We'll see,' she replied, and changed the subject. The family didn't know how to deal with my confusion. Once, on the street, I saw a priest.

'What's that?' I asked.

'That's a priest. Christians have priests, like Jews have rabbis.'

'What are Christians?'

'It's a religion, like being Jewish. In Italy most people are Christians.'

I was stunned. I'd never heard of Christians. I'd assumed the whole world was made up of Jews, Arabs and British police. That's when it was decided to send me to a Jewish school in inner city Trieste rather than the school closest to home.

'But will I have a fascist uniform and be a *piccola italiana*?'

'There's plenty of time for that. You'll have a nice white smock with a big blue bow.' Tante didn't know that it was compulsory for children in all Italian schools to wear fascist uniforms on special occasions. I was delirious when, soon after I'd started school, I got the uniform. But much to my annoyance, instead of the admiration I craved, the family ignored me when I paraded in it at home. Even Berta ridiculed me. Nobody dared enlighten me.

◎ ◎ ◎ ◎

As *Galatea* drifted on silently, I dug my head into Felix's chest and cried. It was a relief when he said, 'Time to turn on the engine and take down the sails.' I pulled myself together, washed my face, put on sunglasses, and gave him a hug.

'Welcome to Trieste Yacht Club,' the marina supervisor called out from the office window as he saw us approach. 'Make for the empty berth to port. When you're ready, come up to the office!'

The tables on the marina deck were crowded with diners. Some watched us tie up, and waved. Flags fluttered above the marina, seagulls circled and loudspeakers sang.

When Felix came down from the office, I noticed him talking to an elegant couple in their 40s. The woman, exquisitely groomed, had coiffed dark hair and a spotted scarf around her neck. The man had a receding hairline, an aquiline nose, and wore wire-rimmed glasses.

'They asked us to join them,' Felix said when he came on board. 'They've just come back from Greece. They'd like to know about the west coast of Italy.'

'OK, I'm ready.' I no longer felt embarrassed by our non-designer attire. Being foreign and from the Antipodes excused us from competing with the style-conscious Mediterraneans.

We shook hands and introduced ourselves. 'Claudio, my wife Eugenia...'

Claudio motioned the waiter to bring two more wine glasses. The waiter came to take our orders.

'*Scampi fritti per me, grazie*,' I said.

'You speak Italian?' Eugenia asked me.

'I did once, but now it's rusty.'

'But your pronunciation…you have no accent.'

'I lived here for almost three years when I was a child.'

There was a long silence. I sensed their quick reckoning. Before their time. Fascism, the war…

'When did you leave?'

'We left before the war, we were Jewish,' I said.

She looked astonished, 'My family is Jewish, my parents were interned for three years in Yugoslavia. They're dead now. I was born after the war. So you went to school here?'

'Yes, I went to the Jewish school in Via del Monte.'

'My father's uncle taught at that school.'

'What was his name?'

'Segre.'

'Segre? Signor Segre? The scripture teacher?'

Felix and I looked at each other in disbelief. He'd heard about my battles with Signor Segre.

◎◎◎◎

After three months' private tuition I passed the entrance exam to third class. I was apprehensive on my first day at the Jewish school in Via del Monte. It didn't look like a school. It was on the third floor of a building, and there was no schoolyard. But I liked the look of my form teacher, Signorina Windspach, with her dark smiling eyes and jolly round face. She introduced me to the class and sat me next to a girl called Fortunata Belleli. 'After play lunch we have scripture,' Fortunata told me.

The class stood when Signor Segre, attired in a buttoned up dark suit and a homburg, entered the classroom. With his heavy black moustache and piercing black eyes, his face looked menacing. He surveyed the class, his eyes locking onto people's faces like searchlights. Shivers ran down my spine. I sensed anger.

'*Buongiorno, Signor Segre!*' The class said in unison. Signor Segre returned our greeting. After a long silence, he signalled with a nod. The class commenced to recite: '*Shema Yisrael Adonai Eloheinu Adonai echad…*' I looked around. I was silent, had no idea what this was. As soon as the recital ended, the class sat down.

'You!' he shouted, pointing to me. 'Stand up. Why didn't you recite the Shema?'

'I don't know what it is, Signor.'

'You! A child from the Holy Land! You don't know the most important Jewish prayer?'

'No, Signor.'

'How is it possible a child from the Holy Land does not know the Shema? What sort of a school did you go to?'

'Just an ordinary school, Signor.'

The silence was tangible. Everyone's eyes were on me.

'Tell me then, you child from the Holy Land, do you write and sew on the Sabbath?'

'*Si, Signor.*'

'And I suppose you eat meat and milk at the same time?' His eyes flashed. My head buzzed. Why these questions? What does he want?

'Sometimes. It all depends, Signor.'

'So you are not Kosher?'

Kosher. I'd heard the word before, but what did it mean?

'I don't know, Signor.'

'You! From Erez Israel!' he bellowed. 'You stand before the class and tell us that you don't know what it is to be Kosher?'

He stopped to catch his breath, then boomed, 'You know what you are? You are a LIAR!'

LIAR, LIAR, LIAR rang through my spinning head.

'I AM NOT A LIAR! I DON'T TELL LIES!' I shrieked.

'Come out here!' he commanded. I hesitated.

'Come here, do you hear me?'

I walked out slowly.

'Hold out your hands! BOTH hands!' He picked up a long ruler, raised it slowly, then slammed it down onto each hand. 'And you shall get this every day until you learn to tell the truth! Do you understand?' Tears of anger rolled down my cheeks. I thought of my teacher in Haifa, of my parents, my grandmother, my brother, my friends…

Signor Segre turned away and continued with his lesson.

◎ ◎ ◎ ◎

The memory of Signor Segre has remained with me all my life. I said nothing of this, and tried to keep my face neutral as Eugenia said in disbelief, 'So you remember him? I must tell my cousin, she'd be his granddaughter, I think.'

'Oh yes! I remember him very well!' I said, and changed the subject. 'We're looking forward to exploring Trieste, but we have to pick up our car from Florence first.'

'We'd love to show you round but we're leaving tomorrow. You'll probably find Trieste hasn't changed much.'

I wanted to see the house where we'd lived in Barcola and perhaps ask to be allowed in. I also hoped to visit the school, but I didn't know whether I could cope emotionally.

Two policemen stood outside the front door of the building in which the school still functioned. Apart from Signor Segre, I'd been happy there. I loved the teachers and got on well with my classmates. But I didn't see them after school. They lived on the other side of town around the area of the old ghetto.

My heart raced as Felix and I approached the entrance to the school, when suddenly, I turned and ran down the hill as fast as I could. Felix caught me, and put his arm around my shoulders. 'I didn't think I'd make such a fool of myself!' I cried.

'Don't worry about it, honey,' Felix said.

'Maybe I'll be OK when we go to Barcola.'

'But before that, let's go somewhere less emotional.'

We made for Café Specchi, where the elegant and sophisticated congregated in Trieste's grandest square, Piazza dell'Unita. I still have vivid memories of Tante and her friends sipping short blacks, their voices ringing with laughter, while I polished off cassatas. But when Felix and I entered Café Specchi, it seemed a sad place. Perhaps it was the wrong time of day. Only a handful of people were there, and there was no music.

I was in turmoil before we'd even reached our house in Barcola. A garage had been added but the pear tree still covered the pergola.

'It must be at least 80 years old,' I said. 'There's a stone table under it. My swing was under that pergola too.' I stood in front of the large metal gate for a long time, then walked up to ring the bell. But I didn't press the button. I burst into tears. 'I can't do it…I can't.' Felix put his arm around me, and we went for a walk along narrow back lanes where I'd once walked alone.

'I guess this is where my passion for Italy started,' I said as we pulled out of the marina, '…but I couldn't have coped returning to Trieste without you, Puss.'

◎ ◎ ◎ ◎

chapter eight

'Can you believe this is us sailing to Venice?' I whispered as we backed out of Lignano Sabbiadoro. I took the helm, and Felix cleared the deck. It was a breathless, moonless night. Stars glittered low above us. The engine's purring broke the stillness. We sat in silence and watched a sliver of moon peep over the horizon, and waited for dawn. At 4.30 a streak of pink lined the eastern sky. Slowly, a golden arc slid from the sea, a breeze stirred the water and caressed our cheeks — the whiff of a summer's day.

'Coffee and panettone?'

The steam and scent of coffee, the texture of fresh panettone, the gurgle of water against the hull and an apricot sky enveloped us in a feeling of unreality. Our excitement was palpable. Neither the flat landscape nor the ugly apartment blocks along the shore detracted from the romance of approaching our dream city. We looked at each other in disbelief. Felix put his arms around me. 'The breeze is freshening, I'll put up the sails.' He finished his coffee, then stepped up to the mast.

To sail into Venice at dawn, as the mist rises and sunrays touch cupolas and spires, is to *feel* Venice. That's when she sheds her grey silhouette and emerges glowing and golden.

How many times had I conjured up the scene! How we'd approach the entrance to the lagoon, see San Marco, San Giorgio and the Doge's Palace, just as sailors and merchants of old had done. And now we were almost there. Above us, seagulls soared and shrieked.

Facing away from the coast towards the eastern horizon, my mind turned to the past, to that day in the autumn of 1202 when the blind, foxy Doge, Enrico Dandolo, had set out with the largest fleet ever assembled on that grand enterprise, the Fourth Crusade. In my mind's eye I saw the spectacle of 500 ships manoeuvring in front of the piazzetta, crowded with people in finery waving and wishing them god speed, and where the crusaders' ships filled the waters from the basin to the Lido, which we were about to enter.

I saw galleys and argosies homeward bound, from the Levant, from Greece, from Cyprus, Crete, Corfu, from all parts of the empire, laden with silks and cottons, hides and furs — goods to fill shops and bazaars on the Rialto.

Felix broke the spell. 'Only 5 miles to the fairway.'

As we approached the buoys, we changed course and sailed to the entrance between the breakwaters. To starboard stood a distinctive black and white chequered lighthouse, to port a tower painted with red and white bands. Our headsail billowed and the engine purred as we negotiated the fairway and drifted towards the Riva degli Schiavoni, Isola San Giorgio and the Bacino.

'Keep going round in circles, I want to take photos!' Felix handed me the helm. Dazed, I took the wheel, left the engine in neutral, and sailed into the milling morning traffic. Vaporetti swept past us, motoscafi sped in all directions, a gondolier emerged from somewhere, bounced off our hull, swore and moved on. I veered to port. The headsail flapped, and the boom swung across with a bang.

'Jesus! You didn't secure it properly!' I glanced at Felix. He didn't hear or notice. Legs astride, balanced against the aft rail, camera glued to his face, he was documenting 'This Is Us Sailing into Venice'.

As I manoeuvred back and forth, the headsail obscured my vision. In the mayhem I hadn't seen the grotesque Club Med cruise ship steam out of the Canale della Giudecca in a collision course with our bow. As soon as I did, my brain froze. I veered sharply to starboard, which brought me into a collision course with a vaporetto ferrying people in the morning rush hour.

Felix, still engrossed in his mission and oblivious to my near panic or our proximity to disaster, continued photographing. I steered to port, then to starboard, then back again. From under the sail I glimpsed people on vaporetti gesticulating wildly, pointing in all directions. I heard shouts of '*In dietro! In dietro!* Reverse! Reverse!' and ignored them. By now I was in a nightmare movie and had lost track of reality. I wanted to call to Felix for help but my voice failed me.

Suddenly Felix came alive. 'What the fucking hell are you doing! There's a bridge ahead!'

'What bridge?'

'Accademia! Can't you see? Where've you been steering?'

'Oh my God! We must be in the Grand Canal!'

Vaporetti listed as commuters hung over railings to watch the drama unfold. Craft fled as if by centrifugal force. Police boats flashed towards us.

'*Via! Via!*' loudspeakers boomed. Now my brain gave up completely. I let go of the helm. Felix grabbed it, spun it 180 degrees. The engine roared. Water frothed. From all sides came roars of '*Bravo! Bravo!*'

Felix was in control. I collapsed. Policemen in speedboats, who had appeared from nowhere, wiped their brows. When I came to, I gave them a painful, sorry look and said, '*Ah, siamo stupidi turisti...*' I remembered the advice we'd been given: 'When in trouble in Italy, it's a good idea to make sure they know you're foreign, act dumb and look very sorry...'

'We are very sorry, we meant to go to the marina of the Porto Turistico on Tronchetto,' Felix explained. They shrugged, smiled charmingly, '*Ah, va bene.*'

I dived downstairs to hide and wait until the pandemonium had died down, then emerged again. With one police boat to port, one to starboard and a third to our rear, we motored in royal procession out of the Grand Canal to Isola del Tronchetto.

One of the policemen recognised our Australian flag. 'I have relatives in Australia.' He beamed and regaled us all the way to Tronchetto with how his parents had once thought seriously about migrating to Australia. I now assumed every Italian had relatives in Australia.

The policemen were angelic. They didn't allude to our stupidity. As soon as they'd helped us tie up to four poles, they revved their speedboats, waved as if we were now best friends, and roared off towards the Bacino.

'Do you think we're the first idiots to sail up the Grand Canal?'

'I doubt it, but we were bloody *stupidi turisti*!'

The following morning Felix phoned the local sailing club at Sant'Elena. 'We're in luck. The guy said that locals flee Venice this time of the year, and yes, they have a berth.'

'Great.' I tried to sound upbeat. Subdued and silent, we motored past San Giorgio, Santa Maria della Salute, Palazzo Ducale, Riva degli Schiavoni. But soon Felix reverted to his old self. 'Cheer up, honey. We're in Venice. We're in the Bacino, smack in the middle where the action is.'

The sailing club was a simple marina with few facilities. Of the two in charge, one was an elderly man in baggy trousers, with a broad smile in a benevolent, weathered face. The second — young, athletic, square-jawed with designer stubble and dressed in jeans — caught our lines and helped us tie up. 'Sydney, eh?' He made it sound as if we'd come from the moon.

'*Quanto tempo*, how long you stay?' the old man asked.

'*Cinque, sei settimane, dipende*, five, six weeks, depends,' Felix said.

'Ah!' He tilted his head, massaged his chin with his right hand, consulted the young man, then said, '*Ah, va bene.*'

'*Grazie, tanto grazie.*'

We shook hands. Then the old man, Lucio, introduced us to the marina's facilities. In his shy, hesitant way, he made us feel welcome. We took one look at the shower and toilet — only a slight improvement on Fiumicino. He continued to supply us with basic information, such as where we'd find the local laundrette, grocer, greengrocer and baker. 'But for most things,' he added, 'it's best to go to a supermarket, like Standa, at the Lido. Things are much cheaper there.'

Back on board, I heaved a sigh. I was in desperate need of a quiet day to get over the drama. Felix, on the other hand, had fully recovered. 'Forget yesterday, we've arrived. We're in Venice! Time to celebrate. Red or white?'

We had been to Venice twice before. The first time was in the summer of 1953, when it was in its early post-war bloom and we were living in London. Although tourists ambled in the Piazza San Marco, there was no crush, and few guides waved placards.

The following time was Christmas 1968 with our two teenage children. It was cold, the atmosphere melancholy, the sky low and grey. Mist enveloped people in ghost-like sheaths, footsteps echoed, odours of hot food filled the maze of narrow streets and canals. And after 10 in the evening all was hushed: most people had crawled into bed. Although native Venetians still lived in the centre, the mood was one of melancholy and sadness, which comes with decay and crumbling walls. Some evenings were so silent and the streets so empty, the outdoors acquired an atmosphere of a netherworld.

One sleepless night during that visit, I stood at our hotel window, which overlooked an empty Grand Canal, and watched a silver moon rise over an illuminated Santa Maria della Salute. I saw the ripples and moonbeams dance on the water. I woke Felix with '…tell me I'm not dreaming.'

But this time we were in 'our third age', and during this, our third summer on *Galatea*, we spent weeks in Venice, away from the hotels, living in our floating cocoon among ordinary Venetians.

Many who had lived in the centre of Venice had now moved to Mestre or other parts of *terra firma*, since most business, other than tourism, had declined and rents had sky-rocketed.

Sant'Elena has always been different from the centre of Venice. It is an island reclaimed from the sea on the eastern side of Venice, a short walk to Piazza San Marco or a few minutes' ride in the vaporetto, which stops there on the way to and from the Lido. Most of the apartment blocks, intended for workers in the tourism industry, had been built in the 1920s and 1930s. It had the air of a quiet Italian residential area, devoid of cars and with only a few motor scooters. A gentle ambience, *gentilezza*, prevailed there.

Sometimes the place was eerily quiet.

Women hung out of windows to call children playing downstairs or to conduct long distance chats with neighbours. Occasionally I spied faces peeping through lace curtains, an accepted way of keeping abreast with the happenings below. Adding to the quiet atmosphere was a small park where old men chatted, women knitted and gossiped, and children rode bicycles and played. Cats curled up in the shade to snooze, or emerged gingerly from bushes; dogs sniffed at tree trunks, raised a leg and marked their territory.

Tourists rarely came here. Waiters at the local restaurant looked surprised the first time we entered. Gradually, however, the locals nodded when they saw us walk past. The baker kept fresh bread for us. The woman at the greengrocer told us what was special on that day, the young woman at the laundrette folded our clothes to save us ironing, and the people at the local post office selected the most colourful stamps to send to Australia.

As soon as I'd decided that I could face the world after my near collision with the Accademia bridge, we clutched our favourite walking guide book, J. G. Links's *Venice for Pleasure,* and made our way to the centre, into the Piazza San Marco.

Although it was late afternoon, the heat was stifling. Crowds in the Piazza were as thick as the pigeons that flocked there. Through the shrieks of children and shouts of guides gathering their flocks, the strains of a Strauss waltz from Florian's orchestra on one side of the Piazza battled with a Liszt mazurka from Quadri's on the other. Tourists shuffled, their mouths agape in wonder. Pigeons took off, spun and swirled, then landed, their heads bobbing and pecking like wooden toys. A pigeon settled on a girl's shoulder, and she screamed with fear and delight. Cameras clicked and whirred. San Marco is a stage with perpetual theatre.

'It's too crowded. Let's go to the nearest church, it'll be cooler there.'

In the shade of the Salizzada S. Moise, outside fashionable shops, groups of Africans sat on the pavement, surrounded by imitation Gucci, Versace and Chanel, eager for business.

We made for S. Moise, who was not the only Jewish saint with a church in Venice. There were others — S. Jeremiah, S. Job, S. Zaccariah and S. Samuel. Venetians had learnt early that a multicultural society promoted commerce. One commentator noted, 'Venetians were not biased to a fault!'

S. Moise was closed. We continued out of the Campo, guided by our noses and the aroma that drifted along the narrow alleys towards what became our favourite pasticceria — Marchini, in the Calle del Spezier. It was packed.

'You go in. I can't cope when the place is packed and there's a lot of choice.'

'What would you like?'

'One of everything. About 20 should do.'

I stood outside and watched Felix point to cream puffs, Neapolitans, chocolate bigne, cream slices, fruit tartlets... Eventually, he emerged.

'How many did you get?'

'Six — two for now, two for dinner and two for supper. I'm sure we'll be back tomorrow. Now we need a spot for cappuccinos.'

The café in Campo di S. Stefano was packed. We approached a table where only two people sat.

'May we join you?'

'*Si, si, s'accomodi!* Are you English?'

'No, Australian. And you?'

'We're from East Germany. I'm sorry, our English is from school, not so good.'

'How nice, you're the first East Germans we've met! I'm sure your English will be OK, but we speak German.'

'You learnt?'

'My wife learnt. I was born in Vienna but left many years ago, before the war.'

'Oh, that's long before we were born.'

'Is this your first visit to Venice?' I asked.

'Yes, this is the first time we've been to the West.'

They were keen to talk, and so were we. We were living in exciting times — the Fall of the Berlin Wall, Gorbachev's Perestroika, the collapse of communism…

We introduced ourselves. Erna was tall and slim, in her 30s, with cropped honey-coloured hair and vivacious emerald eyes. She toyed with her multicoloured Venetian glass necklace. Helmut was a big man, thick-set, with short dark hair and dark melancholy eyes. Both hugged thick white cups of cappuccino. We ordered *due latte* and *panforte*.

'I'm an art teacher and for me it's a life's dream come true,' Erna beamed.

'How do you find visiting the West?' This was not the most tactful of questions, as I realised too late. They looked at each other nervously. Helmut sipped his cappuccino, paused, then took a long breath.

'You know, everything is new for us, it's hard to put it simply. There are so many things we find wonderful, bewildering and also confusing. I think we haven't seen enough to make an intelligent answer. We would like to have more time. Erna has dreamt all her life of seeing Italy, especially the art of Venice and Florence. I'm an engineer, I would also like to see things in my field but at the moment it's not easy.'

They were curious about us, about Australia, how were we able to live on a boat, to move from place to place, to spend as long or as short a time as we wanted in Venice. Did we need official permission?

'It is all so incredible,' they said. 'Do you need a special permit?…to exit? to stay? to return?' These were questions that mark a person who has lived in a totalitarian regime.

RINA HUBER

'No, we're free to go anywhere as long as our passport and ship's papers are in order,' Felix said, then added, 'Would you like to visit us on the boat?'

'We would, of course, but we only have one more day in Venice, then we take the train to Florence.'

'Why don't you come and have dinner with us tonight? Felix has bought enough cakes.' They looked at each other, then said, 'We've never been on a boat where people can live. Yes, thank you, we would love to.'

When Erna and Helmut stepped on board, they were stunned.

'This is like a real home, you have everything!'

'We're very lucky.' I felt embarrassed.

We had drinks in the cockpit and chatted about Australia, about East Germany, about German unification. Everything Felix and I knew about East Germany had come from the media, so we were eager to hear from people who had grown up in that regime and known little else. They were hesitant and careful, and turned to each other before venturing an opinion. They avoided an answer by asking us questions. But the wine thawed their guarded manner. However, when I asked about the importance of belonging to the communist party, I had stepped over the mark. Felix said, 'Time to turn on the barbecue.' We stood on the deck around the fire and watched the flames flare, while bratwurst hissed and spat, and the smell of burning sausages drifted into the evening sky. By now dusk was giving way to a starlit night.

'They're sufficiently burnt, we can go down now.'

Below, paraffin lamps bathed the saloon in a golden light, and the smell of smoke, barbecued sausages, potato salad, Italian provolone, gorgonzola, olives, German black bread, peaches, two bottles of Australian wine and Marchini cakes set the atmosphere. Felix filled our glasses. '*Prost! Salute!* Cheers!'

'I can't believe this! My favourite meal. Bratwurst and potato salad! How did you know?' Erna beamed.

By the time we'd eaten and drained our second bottle of red, Helmut was relaxed and voluble. 'You know, you asked us a straight question: "How do we feel about the West?"... Materially there is no question you're much, much, better off, but you have other problems. We now have freedoms we didn't have before, like travelling, freedom of speech and so on. Of course we know that it'll take years for us to be as well off as you. Big companies are now coming into East Germany, but the problem is they're only concerned about profits at the expense of the workers. I know that a lot of our people will want to move to the West and that will create problems as well.'

Felix opened a third bottle, and the more Helmut quaffed, the more talkative he became. There were many things he'd hated about East Germany — the police state, the lack of freedom of speech, of travel, the lies they were fed...but he feared the future. 'We are not as obsessed with money and material things as the West, but maybe our impressions are wrong because we haven't seen very much yet.'

It was obvious that Erna was more enthralled with what she'd seen of the West. Helmut was more circumspect and thoughtful, with a scholarly air. She seemed more emotional, impulsive. They argued with each other, often disagreeing. We felt their confusion and bewilderment.

It was well after midnight when Helmut rose, saying it was time to leave. We accompanied them some of the way towards San Marco, and arranged to meet in the morning at the same café in Campo di S. Stefano. The next day, after we'd had coffee and chatted for about an hour, we walked with them to the vaporetto. As we shook hands and parted, I couldn't believe that we'd only known each other for 24 hours.

⊙ ⊙ ⊙ ⊙

One of our great joys in Venice was to wander aimlessly, in the early morning or evening, when it wasn't crowded. Here was a carved door, a sculpture on an outside church wall, a small fountain, a statue, a courtyard with a stone table and creepers. We breathed in the aroma of an evening meal drifting from a window of a private home.

'Let's go to the Rialto market tomorrow,' Felix said. I liked markets in theory, but I wasn't happy in a tight crowd. Felix, however, enjoyed the theatre of marketplaces.

For the vegetable, fruit, fish and meat market at the Rialto, we needed to start early. Soon after dawn, boats come up the Grand Canal with meat, fowl of every description, cheeses…

'Don't go crazy when we go to the markets,' I said.

'Me, crazy? Never!' Felix was already looking forward to the banter and badinage.

Piazza San Marco was almost empty when we crossed into the Mercerie and lost our way. A sweeper with merry eyes greeted us with '*Che bella giornata!* What a lovely day!'

Felix asked him how to get to the Rialto. Flinging arms and gesticulating with veined, rough hands, the man instructed us in Italian, 'Go past the first palazzo, turn left, then walk past the two palazzi on the right, cross the little bridge, you'll see a small palazzo on your left, go *sempre diritto*, always straight, then not much further you'll see the bridge.'

It had taken us some time to realise that in Venice every big house is called a palazzo. It can be a crumbling heap, but it's still called a palazzo. We followed his directions and walked into a live painting of a medieval market in full swing. The stalls were already up, shoppers were circling and inspecting, and vendors extolled their goods. Mesmerised by the blaze of colours, the potpourri of scents, sounds and commotion, we stood and gawked. The market was a canvas of fruit and vegetables in greens, yellows, reds, golds, purple…

Felix was in his element. Following the lead of housewives and restaurateurs, he smelt and prodded, tasted and commented, 'This feels too hard, too soft, not ripe…' while I stood and watched an old man cut a melon, offer a piece to Felix with a flourish, then study his reaction. '*Buono*, eh?'

'Uhm, *buonissimo*!' Then he cut a peach…Felix rolled his eyes with the pleasure of it. The man's face exploded into a network of delight.

In butchers' shops, trays of hares, pigeons, quails, boned and stuffed ducks and chickens, and crumbed zucchinis stuffed with mince meat were on display to tempt and confuse.

'The de-boned stuffed ducks and chickens are fantastic,' the butcher assured Felix.

'Please, don't buy meat. It's taking me time to recover from Yugoslavia,' I said.

'OK. Let's move on to the cheeses.' Felix was ecstatic. I took deep breaths and waited outside.

'You've bought enough provisions for a restaurant.'

He ignored me, smiling to himself. 'Now let's go to the pescheria.'

The fish market, an open colonnaded Gothic building, was packed and smelt of the sea and fresh fish. Vendors had spread out their array of seafood, with the name and origin of each item clearly displayed. Salmon from Norway, *polpa* di S. Pietro (John Dory) from Sicily, *cagnoletto* (toothless shark) from Caorle, Prolache crabs from the Laguna di Venezia…Near me an eel wriggled. A boy picked it up, surprising me into an undignified shriek.

'Don't ever take me into a fish market again!'

'OK, OK, I know when I'm beaten. Let's go and have coffee,' said Felix.

◎ ◎ ◎ ◎

Felix was looking tired, my nightly rashes had returned with a vengeance, and we couldn't sleep. Both my arms were bandaged to protect the split grafts Felix had done to repair flaps of skin that had sloughed off. But we were looking forward to a visit from our son and daughter-in-law. For the week David and Anne would be with us, we'd arranged a berth for *Galatea* in the old marina on the island of San Giorgio Maggiore. The notion of breakfasting in the cockpit in full view of the Doge's Palace, San Marco and Santa Maria della Salute was irresistible. In addition, the Regata Storica was to be held the day after their arrival. Felix looked excited when he returned from the hardware store.

'They told me at Ratti's that we can get tickets for the regatta at the Tourist Bureau off the Piazza. Let's go there.'

At the Tourist Bureau we waited and waited for an officious woman to notice us, but when that seemed unlikely, Felix asked whether we could buy tickets for the regatta. Without looking up, she replied in a peremptory tone: 'We have none!'

When we mentioned this to Laura at the laundrette, she was not surprised. 'Ah! *signori*,' her lips were pursed and her arms raised as she explained, 'you must understand, they try to keep the tickets until the end. They wait to get good prices from tours. You must try more often.' We assured her that we'd take her advice and returned to the booking office the following day.

'Let's try our luck with that guy, he looks kinder,' I suggested.

'We're from Australia and we came to see the regatta. Our son and his wife are also coming to Venice especially to see the regatta. Is it possible to get four tickets?'

'*Un momento.*' He went through a door to another room. We heard raised voices from the back. He returned crestfallen, 'Sorry, booked out, maybe later.'

After several attempts at cajoling, begging and charming as best we could, the young man greeted us with, '*Allora, ben'ecco quattro biglietti.*'

'Success. Four front row seats.'

We couldn't contain our excitement when David and Anne arrived. 'Good news! We have tickets for the regatta!'

On their first morning, we breakfasted in the cockpit, in full view of S. Marco, the Doge's Palace, Santa Maria della Salute, the Piazzetta with its two granite columns — one bearing the Lion of S. Marco, the other S. Teodoro, Venice's patron saint — and all amid the commotion of craft on the Bacino. 'How many people have been so privileged to breakfast on one's boat in the marina at S. Giorgio with this view?' I wondered.

On the day of the regatta, we made our way to Ca'Rezzonico, one of the grand palazzi along the Grand Canal, and climbed over people and scaffolding to get to our front row seats.

Crowds packed both sides of the canal. Venice was pulsating with frenzied expectation. After a long wait, immaculately polished argosies and golden barges appeared in the distance, with the proud lions of Venice fluttering on masts. People gasped, cheered and waved as a procession of Venetian pomp — decorated and beflagged ships and gondolas — drifted past. On deck, men and women in medieval silks and brocades, balloon sleeves, velvet hats and pointed shoes, swaggered and waved.

Crowds shouted, 'Hurrah…*Bravo*!' My heart thumped, cameras clicked, movie cameras whirred. What a day of extravaganza. The festivities continued all day, at the end of which, exhausted, we made our way to San Giorgio and *Galatea*. And the noisy celebrations continued all night.

The next day I came up with what I thought was a great suggestion.

'Let's have drinks at Harry's Bar. Breathe the atmosphere that Hemingway and Orson Welles and Churchill and all the rich and famous have breathed. And what better occasion than when David and Anne are with us.'

'Brilliant!'

But how was I to know what a fool I'd make of myself when I asked for cashews?

'Madam,' the peremptory waiter addressed me, his nose high in the air, 'we do not serve nuts.'

One way to keep out the *hoi polloi*. But I gave Felix full credit for laughing out loud.

We were sad to say goodbye to David and Anne. I realised that no matter how much we enjoyed our travelling life, I missed the family. Not long after they left us we put *Galatea* on the dry in Lignano and made for Paris, where we had rented a flat for four months. Not only were we looking forward to the experience of living in Paris, but also to having our granddaughters Emma, now 14, and Jackie, 11, with us for their Christmas holidays.

We arrived in Paris on 1 October. It was a beautiful time of the year. The leaves had turned golden and dark branches were etched against the sky. Our flat in the rue de Babylone was in the 7th arrondissement, close to the Avenue des Invalides and Metro St Francois Xavier. It was part of a four-storey block of apartments with a central courtyard that had been built after the Franco-Prussian War of 1871.

Our apartment was on the ground floor, with French doors opening onto a stone courtyard. The layout was long: the kitchen (every bit 1870s) was at one end, and led into a long lounge with an open fireplace, then on to a small bedroom that led to the main bedroom and an old bathroom. A bare globe, strung from the ceiling, hung just above one's head when you were sitting in the bath. The owner, an American professor of physics, enjoyed reading there. 'Well, that's the first thing we get rid of,' Felix said, 'we're not ready to suicide.'

The caretakers were a Portuguese couple with a large ginger tom cat called Pilu, who spent most of his time stretched out on a long letterbox fastened to the inside of the metal gate, the entrance to the courtyard. With the air of a gendarme, he checked on everyone coming in and out. Each morning Pilu entered our apartment through a French door at one end and paced to the other end, checking as he went that all was as it should be. We tried to bribe him with fresh sausages to let us pat him. But to no avail. He was incorruptible.

It was during our four months in Paris that we learnt to become proper *flâneurs*, aimless strollers. 'That's the only way to appreciate Paris,' we'd been told. We took this advice seriously, and during October and November we spent most of our time outdoors strolling along elegant avenues and boulevards, through markets and gardens. We wandered along the Seine, and paused to browse through bookstalls, ate in cafés, read the papers and watched the passing parade. Once, we spent an entire day at the cemetery of Père-Lachaise, where many of the famous lie buried, and read the curriculum vitae listed on their tombstones. Several Poles surrounded Chopin's grave, holding lit candles and playing mazurkas on an old battered wind-up gramophone.

We strolled into the Café des Deux Margots in Saint-Germain-des-Prés, where *les existentialistes* had once gathered to discuss politics and philosophy.

'We may not have recognised anyone but at least we breathed the air,' Felix said.

October is an interesting month in Paris. It's a time when many strikes and demonstrations take place. We watched hospital workers, teachers, transport workers, students and others carrying placards march peacefully through the city.

At the end of December, Emma and Jackie came to stay for five weeks. They loved the fact that the day invariably started with a rush to the *boulanger*. When they were delegated to fetch the breakfast baguette, they bought two — one to bring home and one to eat on the way. We worked down a list of places we thought the girls would enjoy: palaces, galleries, the Eiffel Tower, trips on Bateaux Mouches...The girls also enjoyed strolling by themselves to shops and markets not far from rue de Babylone.

Soon after our arrival we noticed a small restaurant across the road, at 45 rue de Babylone. 'The people eating there all look French. It must be good,' Felix said. 'Let's try it. But we'll have to get there early. It's really small.'

The first time we entered people looked surprised, but as soon as they heard that we lived across the road, we were accepted as almost locals. We liked the fact that the seating was tight: it encouraged conversation and added to the charm of Au Pied de Fouet. Most people who ate there worked in nearby government departments. The prime minister's residence, the Hôtel Matignon, was just around the corner. Many of the diners lived a long way from Paris and stayed in hotels or in *chambres meublées*, furnished rooms, during the week. At Au Pied de Fouet, they had their own napkins, which were kept in pigeonholes on the wall. Although we never attained that privileged status, the fact that we were almost regulars made us feel almost French. The place was run by an elderly couple, André and his eccentric wife Marcial, who made a feature of being gruff. She allowed no more than 90 seconds to order, and if she noticed anyone pausing to talk during a meal (and most of us did), she'd instantly be on the attack with, '*Pas parler, vous devez seulment manger*...No talking, only eating!' We couldn't blame her. The place only seated about fifteen people.

Some days before we left Paris, I asked Marcial whether she'd give me the recipe for her chocolate cake.

'You come tomorrow at 8 o'clock,' she replied, without moving a facial muscle.

The following morning, she thrust an apron over my head, gave me a bowl and wooden spoon and said, 'Stir! *Comment ça*, like this.'

Then she set me beating eggwhites with a hand beater and when I asked *sotto voce* whether she ever used an electric mixer, she replied emphatically, '*Jamais!*...Never!'.

After our last meal there, she gave me not only the recipe for her chocolate cake, but also for her signature dessert, *Tarte Merangue à l'orange*.

We were all in high spirits until the days preceding, and immediately after, the start of the Gulf War in January 1991, when the atmosphere in Paris changed. The tension at our end of the rue de Babylone was palpable and the street was permanently filled with police and police buses.

One morning they didn't let Emma go out of our gate to post a letter. That same evening we were at the opera when protesters set off smoke bombs and the entire place had to be evacuated. We were worried, and decided to leave Paris earlier than we'd planned. We parked our car in front of 41 Boulevarde des Invalides, and took off to Sydney.

When David and Anne asked the girls, 'What was the highlight in Paris?', without hesitation they replied, 'Smoke bombs at the opera.' Better than the palaces or castles, even better than the bears on skates in the *Russian Circus on Ice*. It was a relief to get them home safely, and good to spend time with the family. But after six weeks we were ready to continue our peripatetic life.

◎ ◎ ◎ ◎

In April, as our plane neared Paris on our return from Sydney, Felix squeezed my hand and beamed. '...we're on our way again. Our fourth summer!'

'Ladies and gentlemen, we are starting our descent into Charles de Gaulle Airport.'

I pulled out my diary and checked the exact address where we'd left our car at the end of our months in Paris.

'41 Boulevarde des Invalides,' Felix told the taxi driver, 'in front of a long black fence.' The car had stood unguarded for six weeks. As we approached, Felix pointed to it. '*Voila!*' The taxi driver shook his head in disbelief. '*C'est formidable!*' he said. We'd left the Renault under bare trees. Now birds fluttered among spring leaves, and the car resembled a bird latrine. Unfazed, we unloaded our cases at the side of the road and paid the driver.

When Felix connected the piece of starter motor he'd hidden inside the first aid kit, the engine came alive and revved with joy.

'Only one flat tyre. Not bad.' He took out tools and changed it. We loaded our luggage and away we went. '*Galatea* here we come!' I gave Felix a hug. We chose a route that took us via the chateaux on the Loire, the gardens of Villandry, and made our way to Lignano and *Galatea*. This was going to be an easy summer. We'd stay in the northern Adriatic, spend more time in Venice, tour the Veneto and the Dolomites.

'Isn't it good to be back in Venice? Pity the old greengrocer has gone, but otherwise things haven't changed much,' I said as I held the torch while Felix did his annual engine check. 'There are some good concerts on. Pity the opera isn't on at La Fenice.'

'Yes,' Felix said, 'but we'll need to book. And the week touring with Giovanni should be great.'

During a previous winter in London, we'd attended a course on Venetian history and art, run by a Venetian art historian who knew the Veneto like the back of his hand. For us, the jewel in the crown was joining his eight-day guided tour. Giovanni Montenero drove us like a taskmaster around Venice, Ravenna, Pomposa, Padua, Vicenza, Verona, Castelfranco, Maser and Fanzolo.

He was a rotund, middle-aged man who loved his subject. With his arms in full gesticulating mode, he rarely stopped talking and photographing. One night he visited us on board and stayed for dinner. He had a love–hate relationship with Italy. He loved the land, its people and, of course, its art. Although he didn't have a good word to say about the Church, he directed his most vicious invective against Italian politicians and big business. Nothing, he maintained, was beyond them.

'Sometimes, I don't think things have changed much at all. Just imagine, I read in the paper recently that enterprising businessmen have suggested building an underground in Venice! And a government minister thought it a good idea. Can you believe it? To seriously suggest in the 1990s, an underground in

Venice! For that idea one needs politicians and big business!' He puffed on his cigar, stretched his legs, filled his glass and continued in full flight.

'Yes, it is true that we Venetians have always been different from the rest of Italy. In Venice, as far back as the thirteenth century, Venetians didn't care where people came from, or what they believed in, as long as they were good for business...

'In spite of all the churches we built, the Church exerted less influence in Venice than anywhere in Italy. The fact that the Pope excommunicated Venice several times never worried Venetians. The history of Venice is the story of a society shaped by people from everywhere, all of whom had com-mercial and financial links with Venice. Armenians, Greeks, Germans, Slavs, Dalmatians, Jews, Turks...All met and traded in the "marketplace".

'As for their private lives, the Venetians left them alone, and never interfered. Each group lived in their own district where they built their places of worship and benevolent societies.

'Some people consider Italian disorganisation and individualism part of Italy's charm. Perhaps it is for some, but not if you need to get something done. Without connections, you can't get anywhere. You have to know how to "*s'arrangiarsi*", fix things for yourself. For most things you need to know a person who knows the right person. We work things along networks. That's how you manipulate and exchange favours. If you haven't anything to offer, you're powerless. Sure, this sort of thing goes on everywhere, but in Italy it's an art form. I live in England much of the time, and it's very different from living in Italy.'

Montenero was certainly in a glum mood. I wondered what had upset him. He was letting off a lot of steam and had already put away the best part of two bottles; the saloon was thick with cigar smoke. But when he noticed that I was dropping off, he looked at his watch and was shocked to see how late it was. 'I have stayed too long. Time for you to go to bed!'

In spite of his moods, we always enjoyed his company.

After some weeks in Venice and mooring off beaches in the northern Adriatic, we returned to the marina in Lignano and toured the Dolomites and the Veneto, often returning to *Galatea* in the evening.

'This has been the easiest summer we've had so far,' I said. 'No drama, and do you realise, Puss, you've had no major repairs.' Felix grunted. 'It was good, but next summer I'd like to move on. I'd hate to stay in the same place every year.'

In September we put *Galatea* back on the hard in Lignano and returned to London for the winter.

This time, we moved into a flat we'd bought to solve our perpetual accommodation problems. We needed a place to which we could return at any time. It was tiny — one bedroom, a living room, kitchen and bathroom. Close to a tube station, it was only half an hour's walk to Marble Arch. From the two front windows of 56 Blomfield Road we overlooked Little Venice, where barges floated down the canal, and from the back window we looked over English gardens. With the help of Percy the handyman, we sweated for three months wallpapering, painting and furnishing to make the place feel like home. Then it was almost time to think about our next summer and *Galatea*.

◎◎◎◎

chapter nine

When we returned to Lignano this time, we were hoping to go a long way. We spent several days there, organising and checking equipment on *Galatea*, then sailed to Venice.

'We'll have to start moving if we want to get to Turkey this summer.' Felix was standing at the navigation table, poring over charts. It was 7 o'clock, the thermometer already registered 29°C and I was still in bed. I stretched, touched the warm cabin ceiling, felt the burning porthole above me, and curled up again. Too hot to stay in bed, too tired to get up.

'It'll take us at least ten days to get to Otranto. Then we'll have to go through the NATO blockade to get to Corfu. We'll need to leave on Thursday at the latest. The long-range forecast is for another *bora*.'

'Right! Watch me, I'm getting up, quick cold shower to wake up. I'll be ready in ten minutes. Let's have coffee and a roll when we go for the mattresses, before the heat kills us.' I squeezed past the navigation table, and gave Felix a hug. It was 8 o'clock and steam was already rising from the pavements as we crossed the piazza into the maze of narrow streets. It was cooler in these alleys, where the sun rarely penetrated.

'Ah, you are here to pick up the mattresses,' Vittorio smiled. He was a slight man with thinning grey hair, a gentle, creased face and tobacco-stained teeth. 'I thought you'd come today. You said you'd be leaving Venice soon.'

We'd got to know Vittorio during our two summers, and each time we passed by, we went in for a chat and coffee. When he'd heard that we were from Australia, he regaled us with stories of his relatives who had migrated to Queensland many years ago. 'But Lucia, my wife, didn't want to leave her family, so we stayed.' He'd been working in Venice since he'd returned from North Africa after the war many years before.

'Angela, get us three coffees! We must have one last coffee before you leave!'

'So where will we find you next time we come to Italy?' Felix asked.

'We plan to retire to my wife's village and grow vegetables. I'll write down the address for you on this piece of paper and you must visit us.'

'San Zannone, that's near Treviso,' Felix checked the address. 'OK, next time we're in the Veneto, you'll see us, that's a promise!' A sharp pain pierced my heart when he said that. 'Goodbye, Vittorio, look after yourself. With luck we'll meet again, and thank you for everything.'

'Are you sure you can carry the mattresses?'

'No problem, we'll go to San Marco and get the vaporetto.'

'Goodbye, and *buon viaggio*.' We shook Vittorio's calloused hand. He escorted us to the door and waved. I wanted to cry. We'd established such a warm rapport with so many people, and each goodbye was more difficult.

I took a deep breath, tucked a mattress under my arm, and weaved my way through narrow streets, squeezing past beaming tourists, with Felix following behind. We bumped into people left and right as we threaded our way up and over a small bridge near Ratti's hardware. The aroma of coffee and body odours filled the air, but we struggled on along the Mercerie, Venice's most elegant shopping street, until we emerged into Piazza San

Marco, and crossed to the vaporetto station. The vaporetto was packed with tourists.

It's easy to pick first-time visitors to Venice. They spin and twist their heads like curious geese to take it all in. The commotion on the water, the near collisions of gondolas and ferries, speedboats and yachts, the blaring of horns, the palazzi along the Grand Canal, Santa Maria della Salute, the Doge's Palace, San Giorgio Maggiore...

I squeezed and pushed to get on the vaporetto, mattress under one arm, with Felix close behind. A local on his way to work cursed under his breath as we came on board. I caught Felix's eye. We smiled at each other in sick amusement. Standing next to me was an elderly English couple with a broad Midlands accent. The woman looked us up and down. I heard her whisper to her husband, 'They're a bit old for carriers!' To be mistaken for aged Venetian carriers was too hilarious to resist, so I said, 'We sure are too old to be carriers!' Impeccable English from the mouth of this clapped out female she took to be Venetian collapsed the woman's face. For some seconds, she was dumbstruck, her mouth hung open, then she gathered herself, pushed and fled as fast as she could to the other side.

We'd been in and out of Venice three times during our two summers in the northern Adriatic, and had spent over eight weeks in Sant'Elena. Our faces were familiar at the post office, the laundrette, the greengrocer, the baker and the delicatessen at the Lido. We knew the vaporetto timetables, and we each had our three-year travelling concession card, the Carta Venezia. When we'd left Venice on previous occasions we found it painful enough. But this time we knew we wouldn't return. Venice had been the highlight of our travels, and now it was time to leave. The notion that time was not on our side was always with us; we didn't need to articulate this. But we also knew that we had never felt as free, and unencumbered by obligations, as we were then.

◎ ◎ ◎ ◎

A heavy mist hung over the lagoon as we motored past the black and white buoy at the start of our journey towards Greece and Turkey. Our last view of the golden city was of cupolas and campaniles outlined in dark grey, as Monet would have painted them. Out at sea, fishing boats drifted on glassy water, some visible to the eye, others only on the radar. We hadn't been out long when I started a migraine. 'I was due for one. Haven't had one for a while.'

'Here's a tablet, sweetie. I've covered the portholes, go and lie down.' I made for the darkened aft cabin, closed my eyes and covered my head with a pillow. Some time later I sensed a change in *Galatea*'s movement. A breeze had come up. I heard Felix put up sails and switch off the thumping engine. Hours later, when I came up on deck, we were approaching the entrance to Porto Garibaldi.

'How're you feeling?'

'Soft in the head, but the pain's better.'

'Will you jump ashore and tie up or shall I?'

'I'll try.'

We made for the pier. I tried to jump but the wind pushed us away. We tried again, and again I missed. A man standing on the pier watched and turned away.

'He can see we want to tie up, can't he give us a hand?' Then I remembered. Of course. He's an Italian who thinks we'd lose face if he offered unrequested help.

'*Scusi signor*, can you help me, please.'

'*Con piacere*, with pleasure.' He rushed towards us, and I threw him a line. He caught it and tied us to a bollard, just as I was about to bring up my breakfast.

In spite of the heat and noise on the packed marina, we slept in late the following morning. 'Let's hire bikes and look around the place.'

'You know I can't ride a bike. It's my deprived childhood.'

'You can get a tricycle,' Felix assured me.

'OK.'

When Felix got onto his bicycle, he fell.

'What's up?'

'I don't know. Can't balance. I'll try a tricycle too.'

When he tried a tricycle, he noticed a loss of control in his left arm and numbness on the left side of his face. We switched to a four-wheeler with a sunroof, but returned it after ten minutes. Felix was feeling progressively worse. My stomach sank. I locked myself in the toilet to pull myself together. 'Is this another Grande Motte? What next?' I wondered. Felix was very quiet. He didn't mention the need to get medical attention. If he'd thought it was necessary, he would have suggested it. So I said nothing.

On the following day the numbness in his face was gone but his coordination was still bad. We decided to stay put until he felt better.

When we set out for Cattolica a week later the wind was gentle. An hour later the wind was howling and we were making 7 knots. Two hours later it was dead calm, the sea a pond. We turned on the engine.

'Typical Mediterranean!' At 12, I went down to get lunch.

'Shit, Puss, the red alarm light's on! There's always some damn thing!'

'OK, switch off the engine, come up and keep an eye on the fishing boats. I'll have a look.' Felix opened the panels around the engine to look for the problem. I kept watch while we drifted. 'It's a broken fan belt.' Felix popped his head out. 'I'll get the spare. Lucky it's so still. Wouldn't have been so easy fixing it this morning when it was blowing.'

I kept watch as a sheet of still satin haze enveloped us, and through the mist, fishing boats and coastline appeared like dark grey ink lines on a soft cream Chinese scroll. In the late afternoon the wind came up again just as we turned into the port of Cattolica, a small square working harbour that didn't cater for visiting yachts. Fishermen sat on decks, some with glasses in their hands, others mending nets.

'There's no room to manoeuvre. The place is packed with fishing boats. Where the hell do we go?' Just then we heard a voice call out, 'Australia! Australia! *Qui, qui,* here, here!' A fisherman waved and motioned us towards his boat.

'Can't see any space there, but I guess he knows what he's doing.' We were in a tight spot and could hardly move, but Felix managed to turn *Galatea*. As we came closer, two men on an adjoining boat helped those on the first boat grab our stays and squeeze us between the two vessels. They took our lines and fixed them to their cleats.

'*Grazie, molto grazie.*'

Five curious, furrowed faces, ravaged by weather, hung silently over the rails to inspect *Galatea*. This was not the first time we'd noticed how differently older fishermen behaved from younger ones. They were shy and ill at ease, their shirts and trousers worn — no T-shirts and jeans for this lot.

'Would you like to come over and drink *vino* with us?' Felix asked.

They looked at each other. '*Perche no?* Why not?'

Felix went down to get a couple of bottles, and I brought up olives and nuts. Meanwhile, the men had changed into different shirts and combed their hair. They presented us with a parcel of filleted fish. 'Very good fish, caught this morning.'

'Oh, *grazie*, *molto*, *molto gentile*.' We were touched. Then we all shook hands and introduced ourselves. At first they were very quiet, sniffed the wine, said it was *molto buono*, and helped themselves to olives and nuts.

But as the glasses were replenished, they loosened up. They talked about their lives, how much harder it was for them now. There were fewer fish in the sea, more regulations and bigger, faster boats with a lot of equipment they couldn't afford. It was hard.

Then Antonio asked Felix what he did for a living.

'I am retired now, but I was *un chirurgo*, a surgeon.' No sooner had he uttered the word *chirurgo* than Antonio pulled up his blue shirt with one hand and pulled down his striped trousers with the other, exposing a long, thick scar. 'What do you think? In your opinion is this a good operation?'

Felix took his time to look at the scar and then pronounced it to be an excellent operation. Antonio beamed from ear to ear. 'The *professore* himself did it because it needed a very long scar.'

When we'd emptied the bottles, they stood up. 'We must leave very early tomorrow. At 6 o'clock. You will have to leave also because you can't tie up to this side.'

'*Molto grazie*, thanks a lot for the fish.'

In the morning we woke before the alarm rang at 5. The fishermen were already getting ready to leave. They untied our lines and slipped past us, as we also prepared to move. Along the horizon the clouds had thinned to silky grey and pink stripes. An apricot ball appeared through the veil. A light easterly breeze swept silver ripples on an oily sea. I looked around. 'It's going to be a magnificent day.' Felix had already turned on the engine. Not long after we passed the marker buoy, we cut the motor, hoisted sails and were registering 5 knots.

But the weather was erratic all along the east coast of Italy, either blowing a stiff *bora* or so calm the sea was a pond. As we moved south, we had a clear view of the Gran Sasso mountain range and the ancient walled villages scattered on its peaks. We pulled into harbours along the coast: Ancona, San Benedetto del Tronto, Ortona, Termoli, Vieste. We tied up in the circular harbour in the centre of Trani late one afternoon. Its marina was crowded with people. It was time for the *passeggiata*.

Small harbours and marinas have a great attraction for people. 'What is that attraction?' I wondered. 'Do the sea and boats spell adventure and mystery? Is it the idea of leaving worries, old life, responsibilities behind? The sea has a power over the imagination. Fear, death, adventure, a new life, escape? Young and old strolled past and looked into the cabin. Were they curious about the mad, the fortunate, the adventurous, the irresponsible, the daring? Frequently, they started a conversation. An Australian ensign always fascinated them. If we told them where we intended to go, they'd often tell us about a fish restaurant there. 'Tell Mario that Giuseppe sent you, he'll look after you and tell you which fish to have…'

Finally, we made it to Brindisi. We had always wanted to visit Alberobello to see the *trulli*, those circular white houses with cone-shaped roofs for which the hills of Apulia are famous. The only way to get there was by taxi, and that was expensive, but we were determined to go. In Alberobello we had a great meal at a restaurant that belonged to a friend of our taxi driver. It had been a great day and we were on a high when we stepped back on board.

Later that evening, when Felix wanted to pay for a drink at the Brindisi Yacht Club, he realised that he'd lost his wallet with all his cards, so he asked the barman about reporting it to the police. 'What did the taxi driver look like?' he asked. We described him, the colour of his taxi, and also mentioned that his wife was expecting a baby in a few days.

'Ah, yes, I know who he is. I'll go and see him. Don't worry, I'll try and find your wallet.' He came back half an hour later. 'The wallet had fallen between the door and the seat,' he said. Then it was drinks and cheers all round.

◎ ◎ ◎ ◎

Felix looked pleased. He'd fixed the cracked lid of the water intake filter.

'How'd you do it?'

'Made a lid out of wood. Hope it works.'

'Always knew I'd married a genius.'

'Is that bacon and eggs I can smell for breakfast?'

'Sure is. With tomatoes, fetta and basil. That's bacon and eggs *à la Mediterranée*.'

'Love the smell of bacon and eggs. Always reminds me of boarding school at 5.30 am after milking the cows. And the smell of basil is one of God's gifts to the Mediterranean.' Felix rubbed his hands as he slid along the bunk to his side of the table.

'*Voila*, the coffee and toast, I think that's everything. Just noticed we're running out of marmalade. Should've stocked up on those great Corsican jams.' The voice of Pavarotti filled the saloon: '*Finiculi, finicula…*'

'Very appropriate,' Felix said through a mouthful of bacon and eggs, waving his hands as he conducted. 'Do you realise we've now circumnavigated the Adriatic. The entire Venetian lake.'

Suddenly, the commotion of boats outside sent everything sliding across the table. A thud against the hull toppled the coffee pot. Felix stopped conducting and looked up. As he did so, I caught a fleeting glimpse of his left eye. It looked strange. A shudder went through me. I dived for paper towels to mop up the coffee, but my hands shook. Felix rushed upstairs to check what was going on. I kept on mopping.

'It's nothing, the wind pushed a boat against us, but we both had fenders, there's no damage,' he reported. I looked at him again. Yes, there was no doubt. His eye was swollen. I said nothing. I had a premonition this was bad news. 'Dear God, please let it be nothing.'

The following morning was cool, and a breeze blew into the cabin, relief from the night's heat. I stuck my head out and took a deep breath. The air smelt of sea, and I tasted the salt. Seagulls squawked and flew in circles.

Felix woke, had a long stretch and beamed. He looked so happy and well. I couldn't avoid looking at that eye.

'Hi, sweetie, give us a hug!' I gave him a hug and a big kiss.

'You know, I think we may well go on to Turkey. I feel fine and if we can get to Turkey we'll meet up with Susie and Simon. We shouldn't feel that we have to stop in Corfu this year.' This was the old enthusiastic Felix talking.

'We'll see. We don't have to plan anything at this point. We aren't in Corfu yet, and it's not long since you were tired and had problems with your balance.' I looked away. I was confused. How could I tell him? Persuade him to look in the mirror? He was on such a high, what would a new blow do to him? On the other hand, perhaps it was nothing. Too much sun, not wearing sunglasses. The thought cheered me. Yes, perhaps I was too pessimistic.

'Honey, what's bugging you? You look so worried. What is it?'

'You know me, I just worry sometimes, usually for no good reason. It's probably nothing, I wasn't going to mention it, but maybe I should. I noticed that that eye looks a bit swollen,' I said, pointing to it. 'I've been telling you to wear sunglasses. Anyway, you have a look in the mirror. See what you think.'

'OK, I'll look in the mirror to reassure you.'

Felix was in the bathroom a long time. I felt my hands shake as I set the table. The smell of coffee bubbling up in the espresso machine made me nauseous. I couldn't understand what took Felix so long. The swelling was obvious. How could he have missed it when he shaved?

Then I heard the toilet flush. He'd obviously been sitting there trying to think. We all do that. Sit alone in a small confined place to think.

Had it been good news, he would have come out and said, 'Don't be silly, it's nothing!' But he hadn't come out, he hadn't said that.

Then the door opened. He looked crestfallen. This morning's *joie de vivre*, confidence and optimism were all gone. He didn't need to say anything. I rushed to him, put my arms around him, but he'd withdrawn and that terrified me. After a long silence he said, 'It's OK, sweetie, it'll be OK. You're right. It's swollen, I'm surprised I hadn't noticed it myself. I'll need to phone Mike Hunt and ask him whether I should return to London. What a bugger!! Half an hour ago I thought we might make it to Turkey.'

'I'm sorry, Puss, so, so sorry. I don't know what to say. I noticed it yesterday but wasn't sure.'

'Let's have breakfast, and then I'll go and phone London.'

He was stooped, his face drawn and lined, thinner than usual, as he walked back from the phone booth. I didn't need to ask whether he'd spoken to Mike. When he stepped on board, I buried my face in his chest, and he put his arms around me. 'Mike's going on holidays, he'll be back in two weeks and he'll see me then. He thinks I need to come back. It's very likely to be a recurrence, and it'll mean radiotherapy and perhaps chemotherapy. He'll decide when he sees me.'

I tried but couldn't bring out any words. Felix said, 'Honey, we've been there before, and we may be there again, but we always cope. You know that.'

'Yes, I know.'

'What we need to do now is to find a place where we can leave *Galatea* for the rest of the summer and winter...We'll be back in April, you'll see. I've just been to the club office. It's the same story all over the east coast of Italy. Since the start of the Bosnian war last year, all the boats that used to be on Yugoslav marinas have escaped to Italy to avoid the conflict, and there isn't one free berth anywhere along this coast. We'll have to get ourselves to Corfu and try to find something there.'

'Yes.' Next to us a group of people were tying up their boat. All were laughing. Even their poodle jumped up and down, barking with joy. I looked at them. How transient, how ephemeral it all was!

We left Brindisi early the following morning and tied up to three fishing vessels in Otranto. It blew 25 to 30 knots all night and neither of us slept. The rain was relentless. We were anxious to move on and get to Corfu to find a winter berth for *Galatea*. To do that we had to sail through the NATO blockade.

'I'll go across to the fishing boats to let them know we'll be leaving early in the morning. Maybe they intend to leave early too, but with this weather it's going to be hell to untangle the anchor chains.' Felix put on wet gear, then stepped out on deck.

'Meanwhile I'll plot the courses and put in the waypoints to Fano and to Corfu. I guess it's possible we may go all the way,' I said.

On the radio, stern voices from French and Italian warships patrolling the southern Adriatic called all vessels appearing on their radar to declare their course, nationality, destination and cargo. I was still busy plotting courses when Felix returned. 'The fishermen and the German boats are leaving early, so we'll all be on deck at the same time. It shouldn't take too long. It's raining cats and dogs, but the locals expect it to stop by morning. They say it usually does when it's like this the night before.'

'I've almost finished doing the courses and putting in the waypoints, you can check them. I'll cut sandwiches for tomorrow.' I took out tomatoes, hard-boiled eggs and cheese — nothing spicy or sharp, no smelly cheese — and started slicing bread.

'Here, honey, antinausea tablets. I've taken mine. We've been more seasick than usual this year. Should have an early night tonight.'

'What would you like for dinner? I don't want anything,' I said.

'You've got to eat something. Soup, something light.'

'Wish it was easier to talk to the kids. I'm homesick. At least when we're in London we can pick up the phone.'

'Just as well we bought the flat. At least we can go back to London any time now without having to stay in hotels or bludge on friends.'

Felix had no problem falling asleep. I tossed and turned; I was nervous. The weather made me nervous, the warships made me nervous, but underneath it all I knew that I was frightened. Frightened of what London had in store for us.

On deck the boom banged and swung back and forth. I didn't feel like getting out of bed and fixing it in the rain. And

Felix, who would have gone out, didn't hear. As I lay awake, I went through our routine for leaving port. Ticked each item in my mind. Then I remembered that I'd again forgotten to fill the thermos with boiling water for tea on the long crossing. I got up, and put on the kettle.

The alarm rang at 5.30. Felix was already up, listening to the forecast. The rain had stopped as the fishermen had predicted, but the wind whistled through the stays. There was a lot of shouting outside, and the clanking of anchor chains.

Felix switched off the radio. 'Weather should be OK. It'll blow, but the wind's in our direction. I'm going up on deck.'

I jumped out of bed, put on a tracksuit and made for the galley to get a tea and cornflakes breakfast. Felix had already prepared more antinausea tablets.

'The untangling of the anchors was easier than usual. I think we should move and have breakfast on the way.' I heard Felix switch on the engine and put her into gear. I came up, collected the fenders and put them into the locker. We waved. All the boats that had been tied up together were moving out of Otranto. We turned on the radio, motored out of the harbour, and set our course towards Fano, an island north-west of Corfu. The wind blew a steady 25 to 30 knots, and the forecast was for *burasca*, gale winds.

'At least it's clear and the wind's with us,' I heaved a sigh. The sea was rough but the waves rolled in our direction, propelling *Galatea* from astern as her bow sliced through the water. The waves raced and rolled onto the one in front, peaked, rolled over, tumbled, crashed and frothed, sucked in by the following wave. The wind sang through the stays.

'We're skating on water! With just headsail and mizzen we're registering 7 knots,' Felix beamed. Spray drenched our faces and wet suits.

'We're too unsteady running. I'll pull in the headsail to a broad reach.'

Downstairs the gimballed stove was swinging and squeaking, in need of WD-40. The fruit bowl was sliding across the carpet, books and cushions fell onto the floor.

'Look! Two warships. They're moving slowly in opposite directions. Can you imagine what it was like when the Venetians were policing this entrance to the Adriatic?'

As far back as the fourteenth century, Venetian warships patrolled the 50-mile width of the Strait of Otranto, demanding that goods entering the Adriatic be taken to Venice. In times of famine they reserved the right to seize food from any vessel, regardless of who owned it. When the Venetian Empire dominated the Adriatic, entering this Strait was like entering a private lake.

Corfu, Jan Morris suggests, was Venice's Gibraltar. Their greatest threat came from the Turks who, in 1480, attacked Otranto and slaughtered all its inhabitants.

Outside, a thick mist swept over the water, and by midday we were sailing blind, our eyes glued to the radar. Every so often either the French or Italian warship came on air: 'This is French warship *Charles de Gaulle* patrolling on behalf of NATO calling vessel moving in a NW direction 310 degrees, doing 6 knots. Declare your nationality, destination and cargo.'

'*Charles de Gaulle, Charles de Gaulle*, this is British sailing vessel *Gypsy Queen, Gypsy Queen*, call sign WXYZ, making for Ancona, carrying personal cargo only. Over!'

'*Gypsy Queen*, this is *Charles de Gaulle*, message received. You have permission to proceed.'

'What if they call us? Can I say that my cargo is one husband, *un mari*?'

'What'd you say?' Felix shouted from the cockpit. The wind was howling.

Then I heard them call us. I wasn't brave enough to play games with a French warship. '*Charles de Gaulle*, this is Australian sailing vessel *Galatea*, call sign Victor Juliet, Five Four Nine Four, making for Corfu, carrying private cargo only.'

I'd found it exciting and exhilarating as long as the visibility was clear and I could watch the waves and see the sky, but now we were blanketed with fog. The drone of foghorns echoed through the mist. Boats showed up clearly on the radar, and the satnav gave us our coordinates every hour. They tallied with our dead reckoning.

But these waters were notorious, at times churned into fury by *boras*. We were now getting a sample of it. The stays continued to play tunes, sometimes mournful, sometimes high pitched, like rasping violins. The sea seethed, sending spray soaring over the cockpit, through the companionway and into the saloon.

'Put in washboards!' Felix shouted, 'I'll furl the headsail.' That steadied *Galatea* and reined in her charge.

'What d'you think? Shall we go all the way to Corfu?' Felix asked. Our speed still averaged 7 knots and the wind a steady 25 to 30 knots.

'Might as well!'

Beyond Fano the mist lifted and the air cleared. We saw sky. We changed course, to sail between Fano and the island of Errikousa. The harsh, forbidding karst landscape of the Albanian coast was close enough for someone on shore to hear our shouts. We saw goats graze, and heard the occasional bleat. As we entered the Corfu Channel, the wind died completely and we turned on the engine. At one point, the Albanian military outpost at Butrino was within a stone's throw.

To starboard we passed silent, lonely bays that beckoned us. But we were entering Greece for the first time, and had to continue to the customs quay in old Corfu harbour. We made for the Venetian citadel and the lighthouse on Cape Sidero. As we neared the port, the docks and houses of Corfu town were clearly visible.

It was still light when we tied up at the packed customs marina, eleven hours after we'd set sail from Otranto. Windswept, drenched and smelling of sea water, we'd covered 80 miles.

chapter ten

In Corfu all boatsheds were packed and we were desperate, until we met an elderly man who repaired boats. In conversation, we mentioned that we had to return to London for treatment at the Marsden. He was stunned. 'I also had treatment there.'

From then on, our problem became Cristos's personal challenge. He didn't rest until he found us a spot. True, it was in a clapped out shed, which we suspected dated back to Pericles, but that no longer worried us. To drag *Galatea* out of the water, we had to wet logs, heave her over them, then pull with two heavy ropes to get her onto the dry. We found deserting her in that spot painful.

The following day, we took an overnight ferry to Ancona and hired a car to pick up our car in Florence. And lest things go too smoothly, we lost 40 litres of petrol in 60 km on the autostrada, but made it to a service station where they replaced a rotten petrol tube. Two days later we were home in London.

I flicked through a pile of old magazines near a window in the Marsden waiting room, and waited. Now and again I looked at the people around me. By now it was a familiar place — the sad, haggard and worried faces; the rattle of trolleys, the clatter of cups; the nurses' urgent footsteps, a patient being called. People spoke in whispers, as if silence was associated with this place. The smell of food drifted in from somewhere.

Felix looked gaunt and pale when he returned from the consulting room. He sat down next to me and stretched his legs. 'I'll need tests before they can decide on anything: I have to come in at 8.30 tomorrow to have a chest X-ray, blood tests, CT and then another meeting with Mike Hunt at 2.'

'Shall we go home now, or would you like to go to a movie or a gallery?'

'I'd like to go home, I'm tired.'

On the following morning Felix had the tests, and in the afternoon an appointment with Dr Hunt. In between, we went to a Sisley exhibition.

Felix and Dr Hunt looked at the X-rays together. I heard Dr Hunt say, 'Looks as if there may be a lesion on the lung, so maybe you'll need chemotherapy as well as radiotherapy to the eye. But we'll need to see all the tests first.'

We held hands as we walked out of the hospital. Felix's hand felt icy. Although it was August, high summer, it was overcast, cold and wet. I had one migraine after another.

'How about we install a gas fireplace that looks like wood? It'll make the flat cosy on miserable days,' I suggested.

'Good idea,' Felix said.

As the bitter cold continued, we read by the newly installed fireplace, and in our tiny apartment we felt that same intimacy we enjoyed when the brass oil lamps glowed in the saloon on *Galatea*.

When all the test results came back, the news was good. The suspected lesion in the lung was not confirmed by the other tests, so Felix only needed radiotherapy. For three weeks,

Monday to Friday, we made our way to the Marsden for treatment. Although he grew progressively more weary, Felix was determined not to let it dampen our enthusiasm for London. Art exhibitions and concerts, theatres…on and on. We were perpetually tired.

'Aren't we lucky to be able to do so much?'

At the end of the radiotherapy, in mid-September, we returned to Sydney for six weeks. Felix had to have a hernia and a prostate operation. He arranged to have the two done at the same time. 'It'd be a waste of time to have them separately,' he said.

Sometimes, when friends wondered about the frenetic pace at which we lived, I had to admit that the only time we discussed our medical problems was when something needed to be done, such as returning to London for treatment or booking check-ups. If Felix was tired, or I had migraines, we waited till we felt better.

Of course there were times when we were depressed, but these passed in silence. We coped by concentrating on the present. We talked about our good fortune. We never referred to life after Felix. I don't recall ever thinking of life without him. Denial? Maybe. But Felix and I knew that I couldn't discuss the subject. It would have destroyed me. Perhaps it was the tacit assumption that we'd either crash together, drown together or go together in some other way that enabled us to cultivate this insouciance.

◎◎◎◎

I was pleased to get back to Sydney earlier than we'd planned. I was homesick, and in need of family and old friends.

'We'll be back in London in six to eight weeks and on *Galatea* by April,' Felix assured everyone.

But we were not back on *Galatea* in April. We returned to London to prepare for another summer in the Med. In early March Felix had the flu and put himself on antibiotics. His temperature was going up and down. Much of the time it was between 39° and 40°C. When he seemed to be improving, we booked our flight to Corfu. We were on a high when we set off to the ship chandlers to buy a GPS and a weather fax for *Galatea*.

The following day, however, Felix started to cough badly. His temperature went up again. Hans, a close friend and general practitioner, listened to his chest. He diagnosed pneumonia. We went to the Marsden for new X-rays and a blood test. Dr Hunt, the radiotherapist and a physician at the Brompton Chest Hospital all thought he should have a biopsy. Felix was exhausted and looked ashen. I cancelled our flights.

Three days later, Felix had an appointment for another CT scan of the chest and a chest X-ray at the Brompton. He had no temperature and was feeling better when he returned to the hospital some days later for a lung biopsy. He discussed the procedure with the pathologist and decided he didn't want it done. They agreed to wait. During this period, Felix had to force himself to eat, and was unusually quiet, thin, pale and tired. I felt I was falling apart.

A week later, Felix had another appointment with Dr Hunt and the chest physician. The latest X-rays indicated that the shadow was disappearing. The consensus was that the problem had been an abscess on the lung caused by a compressed bronchus as a result of the lymphoma. They felt that a biopsy was no longer necessary.

This cheered us no end. We re-booked our flights to Crete, with a stopover in Prague.

During this time, my rash problem, which had started after we'd left Australia, had taken off once more. By now I'd seen dermatologists in London, Sydney, Paris and Stockholm, and none could find the cause. I was finally sent to an allergist in London who diagnosed a rare condition, an allergy to a chemical substance used in dyes of dark or very bright materials. As I mostly wore dark colours, the rash was more or less endemic.

'The good news,' the doctor told me, 'is that you will have to get an entirely new wardrobe. Whites, creams, beiges...' After five years, this simple change solved my problem.

But at the same time my neck and shoulder were excruciatingly painful, and my arm was so weak I had difficulty holding a cup; the shoulder muscle showed distinct wasting. I saw a neurologist. X-rays showed up problems, but he was reluctant to send me to a neurosurgeon at this stage, and suggested we wait and see. We decided to ignore whatever problems we could, and take off back to *Galatea*.

◎◎◎◎

We had personal reasons for going to Prague. I have a photograph of my mother in school uniform. It shows a group of six girls aged about 17, in navy blue pleated skirts and white blouses. At the back of the photograph is my mother's handwriting: 'Prague, War Years 1914–1916??' What brought her to school in Prague? There is no one I can ask.

Felix's mother was born near Prague, and had spent much of her childhood in Telc, a Czech town that is now on the World Heritage list. We took a bus there from Prague and knocked on the door of a house in the main square, on the off chance that someone may have remembered his mother's family. A tall, thin old lady, in a checked skirt and twin-set, opened the door. She looked as if she had been expecting someone. When Felix started in German, '*Mein Name ist Felix

Huber...', her instant reply was, 'Then you must be Tante Ida's son!' We were struck dumb. She remembered Felix's mother and became so excited, she forgot her German and spoke a mile a minute in Czech, which we didn't understand. Yet somehow we managed to communicate. Her husband had died in Auschwitz; she had survived because she wasn't Jewish. She cried and hugged us when we left.

◎ ◎ ◎ ◎

Galatea was filthy but well when we arrived in Corfu. Felix was also well and our mood upbeat, especially after we'd moved to Gouvea, on the other side of the island. Three days later there was a public holiday celebrating the unification of the seven Ionian islands, and the place was festive. Flags fluttered from windows and shops were closed. However, one grocer pestered us to come and buy. 'But the shops are closed,' I said.

'They're only closed for the police. For you, I am open,' he insisted, coming round to the marina every couple of hours with his truck. 'You order, and I will bring.'

At the nearby restaurant a large notice assured us that 'Prices at this restaurant are controlled by the Police'. The marina toilet had been out of order for three weeks, the temperature was in the mid 30s, and the stench was awful.

Meanwhile, Felix, with the patience of an angel, was ticking his way down a list as long as his arm, of things he must repair, replace and install, including the new GPS we had bought in London. I shortened the shower curtain and was doing a massive amount of varnishing. I couldn't help him with anything requiring lifting, pushing or holding steady. My neck, shoulder and arm were too painful. So I took painkillers, which helped most of the time, and ran messages instead.

I started with the customs office, where I had to get a pink slip. When we'd pulled into Corfu the previous year, the fellow at the diesel pump alerted us to the pink slip one needed for cheaper fuel. 'But you're Australian, and I'm Greek-Australian, so don't worry,' he said. So we didn't, and he charged us the cheaper price. But as we couldn't rely on finding Greek-Australians on all the Greek Islands, I set off to get the pink slip. I spent three hours in the customs hall with other people who were waiting for the same thing. It was an educational experience, not at all boring. I established a sense of aggrieved camaraderie with the yachties in the queue and also gathered advice about good anchorages, how and where to get things cheaply, which restaurants to frequent or avoid — a general survival kit.

'OK, all's finished.' Felix was delighted. 'We're ready for a shakedown into the bay, then we can anchor there for the night.'

Some minutes later, as we were motoring into the bay, Felix suddenly shouted, 'Hell, the depth meter's not working! Leaks. Have to go back to the marina. We'll have to get rubber sealing. Bloody radar's not working either.'

'Oh, God, when will everything come together!'

Back at the marina I buried my head in Homer's *Odyssey*. Felix spent the rest of the day fixing the problems.

At sunset, we motored into the bay once more, and put down an anchor. Amen. I felt the breeze on my cheeks, and we took deep breaths of pure air, free of the stench of sewage. The sky was full of stars. There was a new moon, and silence. The smell of lamb and herbs bubbling in the oven filled the cabin. Perhaps Corfu was a beautiful island after all, just spoilt by motorcycles, dust, noise, annoyances, especially in summer... Ron Heikell's *Greek Waters Pilot* advised us to 'persevere until Corfu charms you'. Yes, perhaps next time.

'OK. We're off to Lakka Bay,' Felix announced.

'Not so loud,' I said. 'The gods may hear you and something else will need repair to test your genius.'

Lakka Bay, at the northern end of Paxos Island in the Northern Ionian Sea, is a sheltered anchorage, surrounded by green hills. It was late afternoon, and as a cool breeze swept the water, a flotilla of multicoloured windsurfers glided like butterflies and the sound of laughter from the shore drifted towards us. Smoke, and the smell of roasting meat, curled up from a taverna. Dragging a net behind him, a barefoot fisherman pulled a rowboat ashore. Two women, with scarves tied round their heads, and elbows resting on windowsills, chatted from upstairs windows.

'Our first clear day. No repairs. No officials. Nothing to do.'

'Celebrate. Put on *Fledermaus*.'

It was peaceful when we went ashore, but the day's heat still radiated through the soles of my sandals. Few people were outdoors. We sat on a stone balustrade and looked out at the bay. A cat brushed against my leg. I tried to pick her up, but she had other plans. More cats, in all shapes and sizes, foraged for scattered fish remains, or lay curled up in corners.

'I miss a cuddly live animal.'

'When British quarantine laws change, we'll get a cat,' Felix promised me.

As the evening progressed, people drifted outdoors, oil lamps glowed on tables, and bouzouki music filled the taverna and reverberated outside. It was a joyful atmosphere. But when I turned to look at Felix I was shocked to see how grey and lined his face was, how sunken his eyes. I didn't have much energy either. In the taverna we were the only foreigners, and we didn't speak a word of Greek.

'We really should have made an effort to learn the basics. It was so much easier in France and Italy,' I said. A waiter had a few words of English and suggested a platter of *mezzes*. He presented us with a vast array of taramasalata, dolmades, haloumi, octopus…

'This is the best selection of *mezzes* we've ever had,' we told him. He beamed, and said that the lamb was 'very, very fresh today'. I had a vision of a lamb having its throat slit that morning. Felix had lamb, I had fish. Felix's appetite was in fine form. Just then the owner approached us with two glasses of ouzo. But as ouzo plays havoc with me, Felix swigged both glasses when the owner wasn't looking. A number of people started to dance, waving their arms and thumping their feet. I was mesmerised, but Felix looked as if he was about to pass out after the double hit of ouzo. We paid, thanked the waiter and complimented the owner, who told us to come again and try the seafood platter.

In the morning Felix looked better, but the pain in my neck and shoulder was unbearable. My arm was so weak, I let the coffee cup drop, then burst into tears. Felix fed me painkillers. By lunchtime I'd improved.

'The forecast is good, let's move on to Mongonisi,' Felix said. 'It's only 6 miles down Paxos island. We can stay there a couple of days, sleep and read before we move on through the Levkas Canal.'

'Great.'

As we approached Fiskado, at the northern tip of Cephallonia, a young man waved when he saw us making for the quay. He tied our rope to a bollard between small fishing boats, then stood at our bow, eager to make conversation. Tall, gangly and wearing a long, loose shirt, he struggled with a few words of English and German. 'You know Greeks in Australia?' he asked us.

'Yes, we have a close friend, Marea Gazzard. Her father came from Antikithera. She's a well known artist.' But we didn't think he understood. He wanted to know where we intended to go next. When it transpired that we were on our way to Turkey, he looked miffed and left us for the bar.

'He's much too young to have experienced the Graeco-Turkish War of the 1920s. But his parents or grandparents probably did, and in this part of the world, ethnic animosities are passed on like folk tales, down the generations,' Felix said.

Across from Fiskado in the Northern Ionian is Ithaca, which, according to Homer, was the home of Odysseus. At the top of the hill near our anchorage stood the ruins of his palace, and the romance of anchoring in these waters appealed to us. The next day we moved down the narrow strait that separates Cephallonia and Ithaca, tucked into a tiny bay and stayed there two days, to re-read parts of *The Odyssey* and also Tim Severin's *The Ulysses Voyage*.

When we'd left Corfu and started sailing through the Greek islands, we hadn't realised how different it would be from the coastal sailing of France and Italy. We had no particular itinerary in this part of the Mediterranean, other than to sail towards Turkey. The Greek Islands are at the heart of the *idea* of the Mediterranean. An azure sea and sky, rocky islands, whitewashed houses, olives and pines, gulls, the smell of the sea, tavernas…We followed winds, and put down anchor wherever a village or bay attracted us. In France, Italy and the Adriatic we enjoyed talking to local people. But we found it hard to communicate in Greece, so we spent much of the time alone in quiet bays.

Once, a fisherman motored into a bay we had to ourselves, put down an anchor and threw out a net. He was an old man with a sun-beaten, lined face, in a dark jacket buttoned up against the breeze and a faded fisherman's hat. He sat gazing at the water, as old people often do, content to bathe in the sunset and perhaps think of the past. After dark, we watched him go down into his cabin and light an oil lamp.

'He looks so sad…alone.'

'Yes, he does.' Felix put his arm around me.

At dawn I climbed into the cockpit to look for him, but he was gone.

The days were blissfully uneventful. We moved slowly from place to place. The heat in the cabin was excruciating, so we cooled down by jumping overboard. At night the scene and sounds changed. We watched the moon rise, stars appear and silver ripples on the water. We heard the smack of flying fish and listened to the sensuous sound of water lapping against the hull. Then, when night closed in, it was time to turn on the oil lamps, and later, tuck in under a sheet with a glass of wine.

'How can one convey this utter peace?'

'Write about it,' Felix said.

'I will. If we do it together.'

Navpaktos (formerly Lepanto) is reputed to be the most perfect little medieval port in the Mediterranean. When Venetians commanded the Gulf of Corinth, this was their principal port on the Greek coast. But by 1571, when the most famous naval battle between Christianity and Islam raged outside this port, Venice had already lost most of her Aegean possessions, and appealed for help from other Christian powers. Venice took the brunt of the Turkish assault and the battle was hailed a Venetian triumph.

With its castellated walls and castle at the top of the hill, Navpaktos looks like a toy town. Five yachts and a small ferry were in its tiny harbour. We were barely able to go in, turn and come out. After two nights in the Gulf of Corinth we made for the Corinth Canal.

We had heard a lot about the high cost of going through it. 'Whatever you're supposed to pay, they'll charge you double!' we'd been warned. But we were excited by the anticipation of going through this famous waterway.

'It was £100 instead of £40,' Felix said when he came out of the office at the southern exit of the canal. '...But the thrill was worth it. Now let's pull in to Korfos for the night, and move on to Kithnos tomorrow.'

'You're right, time to celebrate.'

As *Galatea* approached Mykonos, the view from the sea was a moving postcard. Seagulls circled, boats sailed in and out, clusters of white houses appeared to have grown out of rocks. Windmills and church spires had turned this barren island into a tourist attraction. The atmosphere in Mykonos Town was busy, crowded and cosmopolitan, which contrasted with the simpler mood of other islands. We preferred to stay off Ornos, at the south-eastern side of Mykonos Island. There, we swam ashore and sat at a table under a cane awning, digging our toes into the warm, white sand. *Galatea* rocked at anchor some metres away. Only four other guests were in the restaurant. A smart young waiter in black trousers and white shirt handed us a menu.

'Are you from that boat with the Australian flag?'

'Yes. Your English has no accent.'

'Sure, I'm from Melbourne. Greek-Australian, came to Greece a year ago.'

'Are you here for an extended holiday?'

'No, I plan to join the Greek Army.'

'How come?'

'I want to fight for Macedonia. Macedonia is Greek.'

Someone called him. 'Excuse me, I must go and help in the kitchen. Try the fish. It's very fresh today. Enjoy Greece.'

One visit to Mykonos Town, with its razzamatazz, was enough for me, but Felix wanted to go again. 'You go. I'll stay on board.' He was back soon, a little shell-shocked. 'It's the first time I've been propositioned by a male. The place has changed since we were here ten years ago.'

The island of Levithia is the antithesis of Mykonos and different from other islands. Apart from a few sheep and goats grazing, we saw neither people nor houses.

To anchor in the bay of an uninhabited Greek island, where rays bounced off a rocky foreshore at sunset and coloured the water a burning copper; to hear the murmur of waves rolling onto the shore, the occasional shriek of a gull, the whistle of breeze through the stays; to have books, wine and music; to feel the other there, exchange a look, a smile, was solitude and freedom at its most perfect.

It blew hard on the leg from Levithia to Kos, our last stop in Greece before heading to Bodrum in Turkey. We backed into the long quay in Kos. It was packed with foreign yachts flying large Greek flags. No sooner had we tied up than two yachties approached, looked up at our Greek courtesy flag and said, 'You won't get away with that flag.'

'Why not?'

'Not big enough.'

'But it's the regulation size.'

'You wait. The fellow from the port authority will tell you it's not big enough. His mission is to make every yacht buy a large Greek flag. Look, here he comes.'

A small round man in navy uniform with a peaked hat, dark intense eyes and an aquiline nose approached.

'This flag not big enough! You must get new one!'

'I bought it in London at the yacht shop. It's regulation size. In any case we're moving to Turkey tomorrow.'

'I won't sign your exit papers without a bigger flag.'

'Where am I supposed to get a bigger flag?'

'Over there, there's a shop. You can buy a flag there!' he pointed, and moved off.

Felix looked apoplectic.

'For goodness sake, don't make a fuss. It's not worth it.' I tried to calm him down.

'He does this with every boat that comes in,' a Dutch yachtie commented as he passed. 'It's his cousin's shop,' one of the Englishmen chipped in.

Felix was in a lousy mood for the rest of the evening. In the morning he was very quiet. After breakfast he went to the shop to get a flag.

When he climbed back on board with the new flag, and picked up the ship's papers to take to the harbour office, I went with him.

The harbour master looked up from his desk. 'You have the big flag?'

Felix held it up with two hands, 'Here.'

'Not big enough.'

'It's the biggest they had in the shop!'

'I will go tell them to get more bigger ones.'

'We want to leave Kos now!' Felix snapped.

'OK, give me your papers.'

We left Greece in a huff. A strong Meltemi, the prevailing summer wind in the Ionian and Aegean, blew force 5 to 6, and we did 7 to 8 knots with just a mizzen and headsail all the way to Bodrum marina — the best sail in weeks.

'Dear Greek gods!' I said, looking up at the perfect sky. 'Thank you for the idyllic weather in the Ionian and Aegean.'

⊚⊚⊚⊚

Hi Kids,

We're in Bodrum. Alias ancient Halicarnassus, where Herodotus was born in the fourth century BC, during the reign of Mausolus, who built a vast tomb for himself here, thus giving the world the word 'mausoleum'.

The town is dominated by a spectacular castle on a high peninsula at the harbour entrance, built by the Knights of St John in the fifteenth century as a fortress and stepping stone for their assault on Jerusalem.

Our marina is the most efficient we've seen so far, with repair facilities, a mini supermarket, telephones, fax machines and anything you could wish for to make us yachties happy. But most impressive are the luxurious marble showers and toilets, not to mention marble floors with scattered Turkish rugs. The people are friendly and helpful.

On our first evening, we ate at the marina restaurant, under a blaze of stars and a full moon, with an unobstructed view of the floodlit castle and bay. Our waiter, a medical student from Istanbul, tall and slim, a perfect charmer, is here for the summer vacation to earn next year's university fees.

I can't tell you how excited we are about seeing you all in Turkey. Meanwhile, we'll check out places to take you. We'd like to sail from Bodrum to Antalya, but are unlikely to go further. We've been told by a Turk that when God made Hell he was dissatisfied, so he created flies and Mesopotamia. Anything past Antalya, he assures us, is close to Mesopotamia.

> Dad still gets extremely tired, but ignores it. My
> neck, shoulder and tingling arm drive me crazy, and I
> also try to ignore it. The heat is our greatest problem.
> *C'est tout* for today, lots of love from the two of us

Until the middle of the twentieth century, Bodrum had been an unspoilt fishing village with carts and donkeys trudging along its dirt roads. It was now a busy tourist centre, the streets clogged with cars, trucks and tourist buses. Along its long, curved esplanade, gulets, Turkish tourist boats, were busy with day-trippers and holiday-makers. Hotels and whitewashed holiday homes had proliferated, and in recent years it had become a Turkish Riviera for beach seekers and yachties.

In the bay, luxury yachts flew flags from Hong Kong, Monte Carlo, London and the Bahamas; sailing yachts, local ferries and ships motored in and out of the harbour. The water was a froth of wake. There was an incessant hooting of horns, frenetic activity and blaring music. Bodrum was a loud place. But it was the Castle of St Peter, looking as if it had risen from the sea, which captured our attention.

The colours of the stone changed continuously during the day, from gold to apricot, to yellow and ochre. At dusk the towers and ramparts glowed amber. When night fell, floodlights turned it into a fairytale castle.

Inside, this former fortress was a museum, supposedly the best of its kind in the Mediterranean. Many of the exhibits had been recovered from sunken galleons dating from the Bronze Age to the Christian Era. As one local told us, 'For people interested in history or underwater archaeology, this museum is paradise.'

I stood on the saloon steps and gazed at the Castle of St Peter through a forest of swaying masts, circling seagulls and fluttering flags against a clear blue sky. From the boat next to us came the sound of jazz and the aroma of Turkish coffee.

'Ah, that smell of coffee. Shall I go to the mini market and get Turkish coffee to replace the Greek?' Felix stood on the aft deck and looked around, wearing that Cheshire grin that indicated nothing required immediate fixing.

'As long as you remember to call it Greek coffee when in Greece, and Turkish coffee when in Turkey, there's no difference. Yes, I'd love some. Apart from that, all I want is to stroll through markets, or stay put somewhere in a quiet bay for at least three days and do nothing.'

'Done. But how about if I look for a tour of villages before we settle down to read?'

We were in a group of eight in a mini bus, which tore along the dirt road, zooming past walkers on the side of the road, smothering them in dust. But the women in chadors and men leading donkeys continued on their way, unfazed by their proximity to heaven.

'I hope the driver said his prayers before setting out,' I said.

The tour guide swayed from side to side as he walked from the front to the back of the bus, dispensing Turkish eau de cologne into cupped hands. A little later, he offered cold drinks. It was hot, and I fell asleep.

The first village we visited was set on a steep hill. It was famous for kilims, a type of woven rug its residents produced. We walked up a curved alley lined with whitewashed houses and looked through open doors, down corridors and into courtyards where women sat on stools embroidering and chatting. Children ran to the front door and checked out the strangers walking past. In a small outdoor café men were smoking pipes and drinking coffee.

'We shall go first into a house where you will see women weave carpets. After that we will go upstairs and see the finished products.' We entered a courtyard and crossed into a workshop. Two boys stared at us, then turned their attention to their kite, while a little girl shrieked with delight as she hugged a baby lamb, and three chickens ran around pecking seeds. A pleasant smell of farm animals and herbs permeated the courtyard.

In the workshop, four women were busy at their looms. Gentle, dark faces wrapped in headscarves looked up and smiled, while nimble fingers continued to flit across the threads. Each of the women was working on a different traditional motif.

'I shall explain to you the difference between flatweaves and knotted carpets, and point out the traditional motifs, and the meaning of the various symbols,' the guide said, before starting on a long dissertation. But I was more interested in the expressions on the women's faces as they continued to work, undisturbed by the visitors. One of them looked about 16. Was she married? How did she see her life, her future? Did she want to stay in the village? Did she have ambitions to go to the city, to join relatives in Europe?

The home, a basic structure with several buildings around a courtyard, looked as if it accommodated an extended household. A man explained to the guide that in this household they wove flatweave carpets used as floor or wall coverings. It had only been in recent times that these were woven for sale. Previously they had been intended only for personal use.

We moved on to another house in the same village to see women card and spin. They used wool shorn from their own sheep, and coloured them with vegetable dyes, a secret method they passed on from generation to generation. Chemical dyes were cheaper but didn't retain the colour as well. At the end of the demonstrations we were invited onto the roof deck for refreshments. The view was vast and open, overlooking a green valley of herb bushes and wild flowers as far as the sea. A stream of cool air and aromatic scent wafted onto the roof. We sat on kilims, spread on a concrete floor, under an awning of dry palm leaves. A slender woman with dark eyes and pale skin, swathed in a long blue dress and headscarf, circulated with a platter of thin crisp titbits with a spicy topping, while a younger girl with long black hair carried a tray of soft drinks and *ayran*, a refreshing Turkish drink made with yoghurt. Turkish music drifted up to the roof from below.

Felix and I sat next to our guide and chatted. Slim and clean-shaven, with melancholy eyes, Ahmed was a thoughtful young man in his 20s who had the habit of continually pushing back a forelock that irritated him. He told us how keen he was to improve his English, so we invited him to visit us on *Galatea*.

When it was time to leave, we thanked our hosts. The women smiled and bowed. On the bus, Ahmed dispensed eau de cologne once more.

The second village was a warren of houses. We walked past the village square to the mosque. The bearded mullah, wearing a cloth cap and fingering beads, was expecting us. 'The mullah is the most influential person in the village,' Ahmed told us. 'Apart from religious duties, he is in charge of the education here.' The mullah led us into the small mosque, where the floor was covered in magnificent rugs. 'This is the centre of village activity,' he said, 'and my role is to bring people back to old ways.'

Traditionally, the mullah explained, the family unit, both nuclear and extended, was strong. For generations it had been ruled by the oldest male. Everyone knew their place, their rights and obligations. But in the middle of the twentieth century, when people left their villages to find work elsewhere, old traditions changed or fell apart. Within Turkey, many migrated to the towns and cities, which offered new opportunities, education and greater personal freedom, thus accelerating changes in traditional values. It was this rapid social change that was largely responsible for the enhanced status and influence of religious leaders in the villages where people were poor and less educated.

At the end of the tour, Ahmed, unlike many guides we observed later, didn't stand near the bus door expecting tips. He seemed embarrassed.

The following morning, just as we were getting ready to move off, Ahmed knocked on the hull. 'I hope you don't mind. You suggested I drop in.'

'Of course not, come aboard.'

'I can only stay a very short time. I'm going to visit my grandfather, I have a parcel to give him from my father.'

'Where does he live?' I asked.

'In a small village about 50 km from here. Not the sort of village tourists go to. He's very old, and likes me to visit when I'm in Turkey. He doesn't have much family in the village any more. Most of our relations are either in the big towns or in Germany.'

'Were you born in Germany?' Felix asked.

'Yes, so were all my brothers and sisters. We speak German to each other but with our parents we speak Turkish, so our Turkish is not as good as our German.'

'I'll go down and make coffee,' I said.

'It's occurred to me,' Ahmed said, 'that maybe you'd like to come with me to visit my grandfather. He likes to have visitors. A friend lent me his car for the day. We can have coffee there.'

Felix looked at me, then turned to Ahmed. 'Yes, we'd love to. We can leave Bodrum tomorrow.'

We climbed into a small battered car, and crawled along the crowded Bodrum streets until the road took a steep curve at the edge of town. Like most drivers in Turkey, Ahmed put his foot right down on the gas, which didn't stop him talking, while Felix and I kept our eyes glued to the road.

An hour or so later, we entered a village of dusty white houses with peeling plaster, and precipitous streets. Suddenly, Ahmed stepped on the brakes. 'Ah, there's my grandfather, sitting at that café with his friends. Lucky I saw him.' Four old men sat at a table, sipping coffee and laughing. As soon as the old man saw Ahmed, his crumpled face beamed and his eyes twinkled with good humour. He must have been a handsome man once. His steel-grey hair was still thick but his leathery skin hung loose on his neck and arms, his fingers were clawed, and a walking stick rested against his chair. He looked surprised to see us, and before Ahmed had a chance to introduce us, the grandfather turned to his friends. From the expression on his face we guessed that he was showing off the grandson who spoke a foreign language, had soft hands, was well dressed and didn't labour under a brutal sun.

Ahmed hugged the old man and handed him the parcel he'd brought with him. He introduced us as Australians, perhaps implying that we were friends. He translated the old man's 'welcome' to us, impressing his grandfather's friends with his skills as an interpreter. The café owner brought out strong Turkish coffees and sweets. The grandfather wanted to know how we liked Turkish food and suggested we stay for a meal, but Ahmed explained that we had to get back. We stayed for over an hour, then thanked everyone, shook hands, and set off back to Bodrum.

Ahmed, undeterred by the dust and potholes along the road, his foot firmly on the gas, continued to talk.

'My grandfather would like me to marry a Turkish girl and stay here, but all of us Turkish guys who grew up in Germany

RINA HUBER

don't like to take out Turkish girls in Turkey, because before you know it, you're forced to marry them. So we go out with girls who are tourists. But some of the guides go out with older European women who like to have a young Turk for the summer. Sometimes, they invite them back to their countries for the winter. But I don't like to do that.'

'Do you feel more German or more Turkish?' Felix asked as Ahmed slowed down going up a hill.

'It depends. In Germany the Germans say we're Turks, in Turkey the Turks call us Germans. They think we're all rich because we live in Germany. We don't really belong to any place, no place we can call "home". If I could speak English like I speak German, I could get a better job in Germany and then I wouldn't have to come here every summer and be a guide.'

'Thanks for taking us to meet your grandfather, Ahmed,' Felix said, as we stepped out of the car back at the marina. 'We really enjoyed going with you. I hope we see you again when we come back to Bodrum.' We shook hands and waved as Ahmed drove off.

◎◎◎◎

David, Anne and the girls came to visit us for a week, and we spent the time along the Carian coast, in the Gulf of Gökova. The Sehir islands were a good introduction to cruising in Turkey. There is a legend about the beach on Castle Island, in the Sehir group, that associates it with Antony and Cleopatra. Apocryphal it may be, but one version relates the story of how Cleopatra came here to be close to Antony, who was busy preparing for the battle of Actium. To please him, she had shiploads of fine, white sand brought from North Africa to create a splendid beach. Another version is that Antony imported the sand to delight

Cleopatra. Both versions agree that they frolicked in this romantic cove before all was lost at Actium. The girls enjoyed the story. Research suggests that the sand on this beach is typically African, unlike any other in this area.

Knidos, further along the Carian coast, attracts a lot of tourists. In ancient times it also attracted a multitude of visitors who came to see the famous statue of Aphrodite by Praxiteles, the renowned Greek sculptor. This sculpture's particular fame is attributed to the fact that it was the first known sculpture of a nude woman. (Sculptures of nude men had been commonplace and thus of little interest.) Tales abound of how her enamoured admirers came to view her magnificent posterior through the back door of the shrine. Although Aphrodite has long since disappeared, an endless stream of people still visit Knidos.

After we farewelled the family, we sailed on to Keci Buku, a bay surrounded by pine-covered hills. It was quiet, and an easy place to anchor. We jumped into the water to swim, or motored in the dinghy to a waterside restaurant. We moved from bay to bay, inlet to inlet, often returning to the same spot, depending on how crowded it was.

We avoided marinas and bays near discos, but each year they proliferated. Often, a camaraderie was established among yachties who wanted to get away from the noise, and we'd hear via the grapevine of quiet spots to moor.

Anchoring in very deep water usually entailed taking lines ashore, tying them to trees or rocks, as well as dropping an anchor. If we did this in the morning when it was calm, it wasn't too bad. Felix would climb a rock or tree and tie up while I cajoled *Galatea* into reverse without veering right or left. But a sudden stiff wind could make it difficult for me. Once, Felix climbed a rock, fell, injured his knee and couldn't move. At the same time the anchor disengaged itself, the engine refused to start, the wind veered and *Galatea* made for the rocks. Luckily, an English boat came to our rescue.

Some of our favourite coves and inlets were in Skopea Liman on the Lycian coast in Turkey. In Wall Bay, where we cooled off in crystal water, it was a short climb to a summer shack we frequented for meals. Erected at the start of summer, and taken down at the end of the season, these shacks consisted of four posts, a rush awning and a few long tables and benches. The primitive kitchen with an open wood fire was a few metres away. In summer, these 'eateries' sprang up like mushrooms in the most popular coves.

At Wall Bay, a Turkish mum did the cooking on an open fire, aided by her three children under 13 who acted as waiters, and Dad, a heavy man with a rotund belly and a good-natured moustachioed face, who chopped the wood.

Goats grazed there undisturbed, the tinkle of bells announced their arrival. When they were in need of a scratch, a drink or a feed, they came up to the tables and let us know in no uncertain manner what they wanted.

We were never alone in Wall Bay. It was a favourite place for people who wanted to escape the sound of discos. The light at dawn and dusk was a dazzling array of orange, yellow and dark pink; the trees and hills reflected moving images in the water.

At the end of summer we sailed back to Bodrum and put *Galatea* on the hard.

'Our sixth summer over,' I said wistfully, 'but back to our gorgeous pad in London.'

'Yes, I'm looking forward to it.' Felix gave me a hug.

chapter eleven

London was in the throes of a beautiful autumn. The leaves were ochre gold and crisp, the squirrels scuttled busily up and down the trees as if winter were almost upon them, and people in the park were soaking up the last of the sunshine.

We were into our routine of booking concert and theatre tickets, visiting galleries and reading. Felix had signed up for courses in medieval history and photography. I planned to have yet another go at painting.

But Felix had difficulties swallowing. He made an appointment to see Dr Hunt.

I was also finding it harder and harder to use my left arm, and kept dropping things. My right arm wasn't great either. We made another appointment with the neurologist. Meanwhile, we continued making more plans. Sometimes I wondered whether continuing this frenetic activity was a way of pushing aside what really worried us. How long did we have? Felix knew I couldn't talk about it, so we didn't. It suited us to go on joking that one day we'd either crash or drown together.

We had two days in Paris, then set off to Bruges in Belgium on the spur of the moment to test the 'Eurostar Experience'. Bruges in winter was almost as good as Venice without tourists. Its attractions, apart from Bruges itself, were Flemish paintings, mussels, waffles, wines and Belgian chocolates. Not necessarily in that order.

However, these little Channel jaunts weren't enough. A friend who had recently returned from Uzbekistan raved about Samarkand and Bokhara, so we felt we should look into it. I tried to phone the Uzbek tourist office, but nobody answered. I tried for three consecutive days without success. Not one to give up easily, I tried the consulate and was amazed to get a reply. Their advice was to keep trying. I tried twice more, then decided we really didn't want to go that badly.

Some days later, we were walking along back streets near Wigmore Hall and saw a shop window with 'Uzbek Tourist Office' written across it. There were no lights inside and the door was a clapped-together wooden contraption with a sign that seemed to say 'Open at your own risk'. We noticed a man with long, stringy black hair, narrow eyes and a prominent Adam's apple inside. We knocked on the glass and he came to the door. The man looked at us suspiciously, then tried to open the door. After a few shoves he managed it, and looked astounded when we said we wanted to know about trips to Uzbekistan.

He invited us in, switched on a light and motioned us to sit.

'We'd like to know whether you have group tours planned for Uzbekistan,' we said.

'You vont to go to Uzbekistan?'

'Well, yes.'

'Ah, you are very velcome. Ve are a friendly people.' Could have fooled us.

'How does one arrange it?'

He shuffled lots of papers.

'Here!' he said, handing us a leaflet in Russian or Uzbek.

'But we can't read this.'

'Ah, yes, ve must do it in English,' he said. The phone rang. He listened until it stopped, then turned back to us.

We gave him our name and address, and asked him to let us know when he had any further news about tours to Uzbekistan. Then a face peeped out from behind a dark, velvet curtain. We saw only one eye, the side of a big nose and half a heavy moustache. Our man nodded to him. We decided to leave quickly, and agreed that it had been a mistake to leave our name and address. In any case, we felt that we'd now been to Uzbekistan.

It was a bad winter, bitter cold outside. From our front window we overlooked the frozen canal. Ducks waddled on the ice, occasionally plunged into freezing water to forage for food, then stepped up onto the ice again. The tree trunks were bare and black. The gardens and the nursery behind our building were blanketed white and the sky was a monotonous grey. We read by the fireplace. We didn't like to go out, but we had to.

Felix's difficulty with swallowing had worsened. The scan had shown a lymphoma pressing on his oesophagus. He was reluctant to start radiotherapy again, but he knew he must. We had to cancel our planned trip home to Sydney. Apart from that, we tried to continue life as usual — we read a lot and went to plays, concerts, classes and lectures at the art gallery. We worried silently and pushed ourselves, but our hearts were not in it.

Felix had an early appointment at the Marsden. It was still dark when we streamed out of the tube among crowds wrapped in thick parkas. We knew the way well; we could sleepwalk there.

Dr Hunt ordered a barium swallow, a CT scan and bone marrow and blood tests. Once they were completed, there would be another appointment to decide on the plan of treatment. Meanwhile, he put Felix on antibiotics for the terrible cough.

After the appointment we took the tube to Piccadilly Circus to see an exhibition of 200 Modigliani drawings. It was wonderful. But Felix looked tired, and the cold was making his feet and toes unbearably painful. He had also started a migraine.

During the following days, we returned to the hospital almost every day for tests, and finally, for a treatment-planning session with Dr Hunt. The treatment would entail daily radiotherapy to the oesophagus for three weeks.

I felt guilty about my own problems. I had terrible pain in my neck and shoulder, and found it hard to sleep. I couldn't hold a hairbrush with my left hand. Now my right was going the same way. Felix insisted on making an appointment with the neurologist Dr Zitka, whom I'd already seen several times. He was short and rotund, a gentle person with an open, friendly face and a sense of humour. We felt at ease with him. He agreed that both arms were deteriorating and he wanted me to see a neurosurgeon. Felix phoned a neurosurgeon he knew in Sydney for reassurance.

Dr Zitka arranged for a combined consultation with the surgeon, Dr Crooks, at the Royal Hospital for Neurology and Neurosurgery in Queen's Square. But before that he ordered a bone scan, MRI, X-rays...

I had never had an MRI before. The thought of going into a tube, like a corpse sliding into a tunnel for cremation, then keeping still for twenty minutes, horrified me. Felix knew I panicked in the dark or in confined places. 'Honey, I'll go into the room with you and I'll hold your foot and be there the whole time.'

'Is there no other test they can do?'

'Not really, they have to do this. It takes magnetic resonance images of your neck. It won't be as bad as you think, provided you keep your eyes shut. If you do panic, you just have to say so, and they'll stop and take you out. But the lower part of your body will be outside the tunnel so you'll feel my hand on your leg and foot all the time.'

Felix gave me a sedative before we went to the hospital. The nurse was gentle and told me to get changed and take off any metal objects. She asked if I had false teeth. I smiled. Sometimes I thought my teeth were the only reliable part of my anatomy.

'There's a microphone and you'll hear my voice, and any time you want to tell me anything, you can speak and I'll hear you in the control room. When we turn on the machine, there's a loud hammering sound that is unpleasant but normal. We'll need to do this several times for a few minutes each time.'

I nodded. Felix gave me a peck and a hug. I felt my heart pound. I changed into a pale blue gown and then, with Felix holding my hand, walked barefoot into the room. The machine was in the middle. I climbed onto the long, thin stretcher. The nurse covered me with a blanket, then fixed triangular pieces of stiff foam on both sides of my neck and head. I was terrified. Then I started to roll into the tube. I shut my eyes but wanted to cry out, jump off. I could feel Felix holding my foot and ankle.

'Are you all right, Mrs Huber?' I couldn't answer.

'If you're all right, we'll start in a minute.'

I whispered, 'Yes.' Then the thumping started. Felix stroked my leg, my ankle, my foot and squeezed my toes, and made me feel alive. The hammering went on and on. I squeezed my eyes shut to make sure I didn't see how close the tunnel was to my face. I thought of dawn at Smith's Creek and the scent of gum leaves.

'You're very good, Mrs Huber. We're nearly finished with the first program.'

The thumping was turned on and off twice more.

'That's it, Mrs Huber. You were very good, we're finished.'

They rolled me out. I burst into tears.

Outside it was cold, but the sun was shining. Traffic crawled along Oxford Street, car exhausts belched fumes and choked the air with stench, music blared from shop doors, people spewed out of the tube station. I looked up at a blue sky and felt as if a rock had been lifted from my chest. Felix walked slowly, looking desperately tired. A week of radiotherapy had already taken its toll.

'Where shall we go to celebrate that the MRI is over?'

'You're tired, let's go home,' I said.

'No, we can either go to a matinee, or to a gallery.'

'Are you sure you want to?'

'Yes, sure.'

'Well, Kushner's *Peristroika* is on at the National this afternoon. We could just make it, get the tickets and have a sandwich there.'

'Good idea, let's go.' We walked down into the tube.

Dr Zitka sat behind his desk while Dr Crooks, the neurosurgeon, inspected the X-rays and MRI. When he had finished, he turned to us. He looked young and energetic, a cheerful Irishman with a gung-ho manner. 'Dr Zitka has told me about you, and given me your history, and I've looked at the MRI and X-rays. You obviously have pressure on a nerve, which is causing the loss of power in your arms and wasting of muscles.' He paused and looked at me, then continued, 'To relieve this pressure, I'd need to remove three discs and fuse four vertebrae, C3 to C7, then transplant a piece of your hip bone into the neck, and fix it with a titanium plate and screws.'

I lost him. I rarely listened to doctors when they explained what was to be done. I relied on Felix to make the decisions. He understood how serious the procedure was, but I didn't, and had nothing to say. I assumed Felix would know how to deal with this. Dr Crooks waited for me to comment, but I waited for Felix to do that. He didn't.

Dr Crooks then continued, 'I must tell you the risks involved. The worst that can happen is that you end up a quadriplegic. But let me assure you that this has never happened to me.' He paused for my reaction, but there was none. Then he said, 'You could also have damaged vocal cords, but they would eventually repair themselves.'

When he finished, he waited for me again. I turned to Felix. He smiled and said, 'Honey, you ask whatever you want to know.'

I wasn't used to this. It was unlike him. I thought of something to say: 'What would happen if I don't have the operation?'

'You'll lose the use of your arms, and eventually, probably also your legs.'

'How likely is it that this operation will be a success?' I asked.

Dr Crooks took his time, then said, 'Well, if you can stay asleep for four hours, and I can stay awake for four hours, it should be all right.'

I laughed, turned to Felix so he could decide, but he didn't. Again, he just smiled and said, 'This is your decision, honey.' I had no choice. 'Well then, OK, but will everything be normal after the operation?'

'You'll lose mobility in your neck. Looking up, down or sideways will be difficult, but your arms will gradually regain their strength. But I guarantee your neck will be OK in a gale force 8.'

'You won't catch me out in a gale force 8. Not if I can help it. But if I can't look up, how will I see the top of the mast?'

'You can lie flat on deck and look up.'

'Good idea. So that solves that. How long before we can go back to the boat?'

'In six weeks, two months.'

I was cheerful when we left. The decision had been made. On most occasions I'm an optimist, and anyway, I had no alternative. 'If we can get back to the boat in two months, then that's not too bad. I can lie on the deck to look up at the mast, but I can't very well lie on the floor to look at the ceiling in the Sistine Chapel.'

'I'll get you a big mirror, plenty of art experts do that…Now then, where do we go for lunch?'

It was only much later that I found out how worried Felix had been. He had chosen not to tell me how serious this operation was in order not to panic me, especially as there was no alternative.

As promised, I stayed asleep for four hours during the operation, and Dr Crooks stayed awake for four hours, and all went according to plan.

Felix had his last session of radiotherapy the day before my operation. He looked exhausted, not only from his treatment, but also because of his concern for me. My first night after the operation was a nightmare. I couldn't breathe properly. The special nurse Felix had arranged didn't know how to work the oxygen cylinder. She also spent much of the night studying for an exam. I was hysterical when Felix came to visit the following morning.

'Puss, I can't breathe. Will you stay with me tonight?'

'Of course I'll stay. I'll sit here and pretend we're on the London to Bangkok leg. I'll ask sister if that's OK.'

When he asked the head nurse, she said, 'Dr Huber, you do realise this is highly irregular, but you may. Just this time.' I thought of the nurses at the Guy de Chauliac in Montpellier, where they had organised a stretcher for me.

Exhausted from the radiotherapy and the cough, Felix sat up all night and helped me breathe with the oxygen cylinder. On the third day, my breathing had improved. But the adhesive they used to glue monitors to my head during the operation was driving me crazy.

'I feel as itchy as a mangy dog. I can't get a comb through my hair!'

'Let me try and wash it off.'

Felix tried soap and water, eau de cologne and methylated spirits but nothing worked. The nursing staff had no bright ideas. Finally, he tried nail polish remover. It worked.

'Ah, that's better,' I said.

Felix laughed. It was good to see him laugh.

'I smell of acetone. It's making me sick, I have to wash my hair.'

'I'll bring your shampoo and hair drier. We can have a go in the bath.'

Next day, like naughty children, we crept into the bathroom. I knelt in the bath while Felix held the shower hose over my head, shampooed my hair, then dried it.

'Quick, before one of the nurses sees us and I get expelled!'

On the fifth day I was back home with a new neck and a collar I had to wear for six weeks.

During the following weeks, I was in a lot of pain. Felix fed me painkillers.

'Puss, you look exhausted. Your cough, the radiotherapy, my operation. I feel so guilty. You're doing all the cooking, the washing, the housework...'

'I'll be OK. You're improving, a bit slower than we expected, but you're walking much better, less pain in your hip, and if Mike Hunt tells me that my last tests are all clear, we'll celebrate.'

When Felix came home from his next appointment, he beamed. 'Tests are all clear!'

'So how will we celebrate?'

'How about driving to Wales, to the Hay-on-Wye Literary Festival next month. Also, there's a great performance of *Eugen Onegin* in Glyndebourne.'

'It's "yes" to both.' I was enthusiastic.

chapter twelve

During those cold months in London, the future looked dark and I sometimes wondered how we'd continue. But we did, and we were back in Bodrum in late June for our seventh summer in the Mediterranean.

Felix made a list of items that needed repair. 'Eighteen!' he announced. He worked on *Galatea* all day. The GPS didn't work, the hot-water tank leaked, the plastic sides of the bimini (the cover over the cockpit) had to be replaced, we needed three new batteries, the anchor chain was caught in the tube, the anchor winch was broken…

'The carpet needs to be replaced.'

'OK,' Felix said, 'that's your department.'

After ten days of preparations, we were ready to take off.

The day before we left, Ali, the mechanic who had been helping Felix, came for coffee and a chat. He stirred sugar into his coffee and talked about his life, his village and his family.

'…My father worked hard. He sold the crops he bought from peasants. That's how he made money. Accumulating a lot of money gave him influence in our village. At the last elections my father made sure that 400 people voted for the party.

'My mother died five years ago. My father doesn't work any more. He lives with my sister and her three children. In the old days, a woman went to live in the house of her mother-in-law. My sister first lived with her husband's family, and she was a slave to her mother-in-law. But today things are different. Her husband is now in Germany and she lives with our father and feels more free. It's better for her. My wife and I live by ourselves in Bodrum. We've only been married for a year.

'My father still has much respect and honour because he is old. When he was young, people in the village knew how to make and fix everything they needed. Older men could teach younger men. Today, everyone buys many of these things, so young men don't know how to make things. When I will be old, I will not have so much respect and honour like my father. I'll only have respect and honour if I have a lot of money. In Australia, old people have honour?'

'It's hard to say. In Australia most people live in big cities like Istanbul, so it's different from your old village life.'

Ali finished his coffee and stood up. We shook hands and he wished us a good trip, adding, 'Come and see me when you get back. Enjoy your sailing!'

'My fig deprivation is really bad,' I told Felix. 'I know we checked out every shop and market for figs in Bodrum before we left, but they may have some here.'

We had put down anchor in Palamut, a small hamlet with a white beach, and we were the only boat there. The scent of pines wafted in the breeze. A group of Turkish gypsies camped on a hill above the shore.

'Let's row in and ask,' Felix said. The shopkeepers smiled, shook their heads and told us that the fig season was over, but '…you may find some in Rhodes.'

'Problem is we're not going to Rhodes.' We rowed back to *Galatea*.

The sea was an orange velvet at sunset. From the beach, the aroma of cooking meat drifted towards us. It was still early, but we were tired, and the rhythmic sound of music from the gypsy camp rocked us to sleep.

Squawking gulls woke us at dawn. On the hill above the beach where the gypsies had spent the night, a plume of smoke streaked into a misty porcelain sky. We sniffed a faint smell of smoke and coffee. It was early, still cool, and our deck was covered in dew. We heard a motor boat putter into the bay. Two fishermen were returning from a night at sea. Their port and starboard lights were still aglow, and the soft sound of Turkish music drifted from their cabin.

Felix checked the weather fax, then looked at the sky. 'It's going to be a brilliant day.' We had coffee and toast in the cockpit, then pulled up anchor and set the headsail and mizzen. With one hand on the wheel and the other holding binoculars, Felix scoured the landscape for fig trees. 'Look, fig trees on the hill above that inlet. The place looks deserted, but maybe there are still some figs on the trees, if birds haven't got them. You never know.' He made for the shore.

As we approached the head of the inlet, we noticed a boat tied up to a small wooden pier, flying a flag we didn't recognise. On the hill above was a burnt-out ruin of a house. Two boys sat on the deck clutching fishing lines while a man was absorbed with something on the boom. When he heard us approach, he turned and indicated that we could tie up alongside his boat. We strung out fenders, threw him our lines and made fast.

'Thank you.'

The man was about 40, his face and hands were smooth and lean; it was obvious he didn't belong to the sea. His attire and that of the boys was 'casual vacation'. Shortly after we tied up, the boys, aged about 10 and 12, started an angry yelling match. Dad turned to them and shouted, and suddenly the scene was out of control.

From the gesticulation I guessed the battle was over a large can that the younger boy had knocked, freeing an army of live crabs now making a dash to freedom. The other boy exploded, ran after them with a knife and tried to stab them. When this proved a useless exercise, he picked up as many as he could and pulled out their legs to stop them running.

'I think I'm going to be sick. Let's anchor out in the bay.'

We untied our lines and left them to it.

'What's the time?' I asked.

'One o'clock,' Felix answered, then added, 'What about we go to Rhodes to look for figs, and stay there a few days?'

'But we decided to go to Bozuk Buku and Marmaris!'

'Says who? If we change course now, we'll get there in a couple of hours.'

'OK, but Rhodes is in Greece. What about Greek customs?'

'Let's worry about it when we get there.'

On a beautiful summer's day we passed between two bronze deer guarding the entrance once straddled by the Colossus of Rhodes. We tied up near the entrance, under the fortress of Aghios Nikolaos and the medieval windmills.

Two young couples tied up next to us took our lines and greeted us with 'G'day!' The boys were New Zealanders, the girls Australians. They were enthusiasts in a clapped out 30-year-old boat and referred to themselves as 'sailing amateurs'. They had little equipment. Not such a bad thing, I thought. It must save a lot of repairs.

'Aren't we lucky. A berth in this crowded marina,' I said to Felix.

'Don't get so excited, here's a bloke making straight for us.'

'What bloke?'

'Just wait, here he is.'

'You come to stay how long?' He was small, leathery-skinned, with an aggressive tone.

'Two or three days.'

'You must see port police with passport, customs, health, immigration.'

'OK, where are they?'

'Will take you two to three days to fix,' he paused, and waited for our reaction.

'Does it have to take all that time?'

'If I do this, it will take only two hours.'

'How much?'

'Twenty-five thousand drachmas.'

Felix took his time. The man was irritated. After a while Felix said 'OK' and handed over our passports and ship's papers.

'I come back in two hours.' No smile. He trotted off.

'That's £70. If I tried to fix the papers, they'd make damn sure it'd take three days,' said Felix.

'Oh, forget it. Enjoy the thrill. Three hours ago we had no idea we'd be in Rhodes!'

'OK, put on your *chapeau rouge* and let's go into town. I'm starved.'

We walked into the walled city. It hummed with activity and people. We went into the main square, and decided on an upstairs restaurant, with a view over the action. We ordered prawns and beer. Felix's appetite was in fine form.

'Do you have figs?' I asked the waiter.

'Oh, madam, since last week no more figs.'

'Never mind, it was worth coming,' I assured Felix. 'To find ourselves here so unexpectedly, that's what I call the joys of freedom.'

Rhodes is a garden island, often compared to Capri. When Tiberius heard about the beauty of Rhodes, he decided to see for himself; in 6 BC he retired there for a time. In 1522, with a force of 100 000, Suleiman I battled 650 knights and their supporters for five months, until the knights capitulated. Turkey ruled Rhodes for almost four centuries until 1912, when Italy occupied the island. In the 1930s, Italians restored the castle and the old medieval walled town to their former glory. In 1947, Rhodes was ceded to Greece. All these influences have left their mark.

We walked through the Palace of Knights of Rhodes, the Street of Knights, Socrates' Street, Suleiman Mosque and the Square of Jewish Martyrs. Two thousand Jews, who had lived in Rhodes, were deported to Auschwitz in 1944. We spent three days in Rhodes before heading back along the Turkish coast to a rendezvous with our daughter Julie and a friend.

After a long absence, we entered Skopea Liman in Turkey. We made for Göcek at the head of the bay. The small square near the marina was now paved, and there was a new telephone booth and a new laundry run by a returnee from Germany.

I was too lazy to go to the luxurious showers on shore and instead had a cold shower on board. While under the shower, it occurred to me to wash my underwear. Soon there was knocking on the hull. I emerged to find a bulky, balding, angry man with a face like a prune, dressed in a tight suit and tie. He barked Turkish at me. I hadn't a clue what he was talking about. A young man from the marina who spoke English came to my aid.

'He says that you have been washing up.'

'I haven't been near the sink, I've just had a shower.'

'He says you must have been washing up, he saw the detergent flow out.'

'I'm telling you. I have not been near the sink.' The man continued to shout. Suddenly it occurred to me. The 'detergent' must have been the soap from the underwear.

'Oh yes, I washed two pieces of underwear, that's all.' The young man was embarrassed by the tirade or perhaps my mention of underwear, and tried to placate the man.

'He says that you know you are not allowed to have soap running out into the bay. You must do all the washing in the washrooms ashore. I'm sorry he's so angry.'

'Well, I'm sorry too.'

'The problem is that he is the new mayor. He says that you must pay the fine.'

'What's the fine?'

'One million Turkish lira.'

'What!?'

'I've tried to tell him that you made a mistake, you didn't mean to have detergent flow into the bay, that you always wash on shore. But he needs to show that he's serious about keeping the bay clean. You must understand, he was elected mayor yesterday and must show that he's important.'

'But that's £200!'

'Yes, unfortunately we can't change that. Last year a man emptied diesel into the bay, couldn't pay the big fine and lost his boat.'

I was aghast, and looked at Felix. He looked at me. 'You sure could have bought some sexy underwear for that, but I guess that's why Turkish waters are so clean.'

As soon as we had hugged and greeted the girls, we made for Wall Bay and rowed ashore to our favourite shack restaurant. The same Turkish mum and dad were there. Mum was still stoking the fire, Dad was still collecting the wood, the goats still needed a scratch or a feed. We recognised one of their girls from the previous year, and her smile was as welcoming as ever. She had grown several centimetres. I wanted to ask where her two siblings were, but we still couldn't communicate. In the evening, thin clouds dimmed the stars and a new moon. The next morning the shore was a delicate Japanese-style landscape hidden in a veil of mist.

In Kalkan we spent hours in a carpet shop that smelt of wool and was owned by a Swiss woman with lively blue eyes and her husband, an athletic Turk with straight black hair and a gentle manner. They plied us with cups of Turkish coffee, and with endless patience explained the differences between various styles of weaves. Julie bought two kilims, or flatweaves, and we bought four. When we tore ourselves away from the carpets, we sailed into Kas, at the foot of steep green slopes. Like many villages along this coast, Kas had been Greek until 1922. Behind the village were many Lycian rock tombs. When spotlights shone on them after dark they looked like glow-worms.

Nearby is the Greek island of Kastelloritzo, a melancholy place. A notice over one door read: 'The Sydney Club'. Early in the twentieth century the island had a population of 20 000, but at the time of our visit, only a couple of hundred lived there. Many had migrated to Australia. The houses looked forlorn and unkempt. Apart from some renovating financed by money from abroad, little happened there. Returnees visited, and a few tourists. In the Blue Grotto, the flitting colours were like stained-glass windows. We walked into a restaurant where the owner went out of his way to make Australians welcome.

Back along the coast, we took a bus to Demre (ancient Myra) to see the tombs chiselled into the mountain, the amphitheatre and the church of St Nicholas. Some claimed that St Nicholas was the original Santa Claus, who had insisted that his generosity remain anonymous. That's why he dropped a bag of gold down the chimney of a poor family whose daughters were drying their stockings by the fire. The gold landed straight into the stockings, and so the myth of the Christmas stocking started. That's how the story runs in Demre.

Soon after, it was time for Julie and her friend to leave us. I found it hard to wave them goodbye.

'So,' Felix said, 'do we now go to Cappadocia?'

'You bet.' Cappadocia is known as the Cradle of Civilization in Turkey.

We flew to Ankara, then made for the bus terminal. A uniformed official helped us find the bus to Urgup, the centre of the Anatolian plains.

'It takes five hours to get there,' he said.

We were the only foreigners on the full bus. The rest were Turks travelling to various stops along the way. We passed tumbledown houses that looked unstable, perched on top of each other, built on what looked like mud heaps. It was much poorer than anything we'd seen along the coast. The conductor came around with a bottle of sweet-smelling cologne every hour, as our carpet-tour guide Ahmed had done, pouring it into cupped hands so passengers could apply it to their face and neck. Some people shut their eyes and snoozed, others opened a newspaper or stared out the window as we bumped along. After two hours my neck was excruciatingly painful. I'd forgotten my support collar.

'Remember how Dr Crooks assured me that my neck could stand a force 8 gale?' I said to Felix. 'Well, that may be true, but he didn't warn me about Turkish buses.'

The countryside was very different from the coast. The landscape was treeless but most was tilled. We flitted past villages with mud houses and minarets, groups of men sitting in small cafés, children waving by the roadside, peasants leading mules and women walking straight as rods with bundles of faggots on their heads. We heard muezzins' calls to prayer.

Finally, we arrived in Urgup. The next day we drove by taxi to the Göreme region, known in ancient times as Cappadocia, to see its unique formations. The exotic shapes that cover this landscape are the result of thousands of years of volcanic activity. The scattered ashes and lava, battered by wind and rain, affected by erosion and fluctuations in temperature, formed countless shapes, such as the 'fairy chimneys' — pyramidal, pointed, conical with protective caps — variously described as a lunar landscape, a sorcerer's creation and imaginary fairytale drawings.

People had lived in these tufa homes, dug into the landscape, until the 1950s, when the area was declared a national park.

The 'underground city' of Derinkuyu was discovered by chance and opened to the public in 1965. Here people lived in eleven underground levels, where they also worshipped in churches and studied in monasteries. I walked down two levels then escaped back to the open air. Felix braved it down as far as he was allowed, to the church at the eighth level. There are said to be hundreds of other such underground cities in Cappadocia. For Christians these were shelters against Arab raiders. The variation of colours added a touch of the fantastical. Depending on the brightness of the light and the hour of day, shades of orange, pink, grey, beige and white enveloped the ochre-coloured structures.

'What an extraordinary place,' Felix said.

'Yes, even worth a lousy neck.'

◎ ◎ ◎ ◎

Back in Antalya, we now prepared to leave for Cyprus where we intended to leave *Galatea* for the winter. The gales started on the day we'd planned to set off. Force 7 to 9 winds raged over the entire Aegean, extending as far as Antalya. They raged for five days. On 10 October 1994, I entered in my diary: 'The worst storm this marina has ever experienced. Hail, wind from south-east. Several fender covers ripped. Closed all hatches. Looks as if we'll be here at least two more days. Forecasts not hopeful.'

'At least this tests your waterproofing,' I said to Felix. 'No leaks. It's perfect, Puss.'

We listened to six forecasts a day, starting with the 6.30 am broadcast from Athens. The weather fax transmissions from Offenbach in Germany and Rota in Spain gave us maps on the computer screen. Felix became as addicted to these as some do to pinball machines. On 14 October, the gales and storms were clearly subsiding and the forecast for the 16th was for 'weather overcast, winds 4 to 5, seas moderate, visibility moderate'.

'Couldn't have better than that,' was Felix's response. I could think of 'better than that' — 'weather clear, winds 3 to 4, seas slight, visibility good'.

After such gales in the Aegean, and storms elsewhere, we expected several days of heavy Mediterranean swell. If this were to become too unpleasant, we decided, we would turn back and make for Kemer. But — and herein lay one virtue in this unscheduled delay — we would have a full moon.

We thanked the staff of the Antalya marina, waved goodbye to our neighbours, and cast off at 8 am to ensure we would reach Paphos in daylight. The 157-mile crossing would take us 24 to 26 hours. It was a bright, sunny, windless morning as we backed out of our berth.

We had prepared for all the contingencies of an overnight crossing, and settled back for a relatively lazy day. Felix was at the helm. We breathed in the pristine air, the fresh smell that comes after torrential downpours, heard the chirping of birds after days of gales, felt the warmth of the sun and focused our gaze for one last time on the vast Lycian mountain range that fringed the west side of the Gulf of Antalya. Orange rays pierced the veil of morning mist and a kaleidoscope of colours quivered over the jagged mountains as we sailed on in silence out of the Gulf.

Then we started our usual routine. We entered our position on the chart every two hours, and made sure the dead reckoning matched the GPS position. We were in a relaxed mood and anticipated a pleasant night. It was not until lunchtime, when we were outside the shelter of the Gulf of Antalya, that we started to feel the swell, although at this stage it wasn't bad. But what did start to worry us was a clear storm we saw on the radar, about 32 miles ahead. Not long afterwards, we noticed that a large ferry 15 miles ahead, also bound for Cyprus, had changed course. We concluded that they had also seen the storm and wanted to avoid it.

We changed course several times over the next few hours. At 3.30 pm we saw lightning in the distance and heard thunder. We were well out of the Gulf of Antalya, in a very heavy swell, but it didn't occur to us to turn back. *Galatea* was under mizzen, headsail and engine, averaging 7 to 8 knots. Much of the time one of us was at the helm while the other was glued to the radar. We had never seen storms so clearly outlined before. Like blobs of ink in a Rorschach test, the storms were forming and reforming in an arc several miles ahead of us. There was no way we could avoid going through them.

By 5.30 pm it was pitch dark. Black clouds hid the moon and we were sailing inexorably into the eye of a storm. *Galatea* was pounded by a turbulent swell that whipped waves and froth onto the decks. The winds, which were now funnelling from all directions and sucking us into the centre of the storms, tore the mizzen and partially unfurled the headsail. We ploughed on under engine, with just enough sail to steady the roll.

Meanwhile, the westerly swell, which had been tolerable, now curled and frothed and pushed us obliquely. I felt the bow being pushed to port, and the stern to starboard. The motion was so strong it tugged at my safety harness. Then, when the clouds parted, a dazzling, stately moon appeared, encircled by glittering stars. The wind had suddenly died down, and all around was relatively quiet, but the swell continued to pound us.

Before I started my 8 pm to midnight watch, we checked the radar together, and saw only one storm on the screen, about 16 miles to starboard. Felix then went down to sleep. I was reasonably happy to be on my own in our cosy, enclosed cockpit. Soon after Felix had gone off-watch, however, the lightning and thunder started again. It felt close, and was coming from all sides. The moon and stars had disappeared, and on checking the radar I noticed that we were in the centre of a necklace strung with irregular storms.

I woke Felix. It was hard to know which storm to negotiate; we were being pounded by rain, wind and sea. Thick shafts of lightning, ceaseless explosions of fireworks from all directions, plummeted vertically into the sea and lit up a black sky. One ominous cloud rose like a tree trunk out of the raging sea and spread into a vast mushroom, simulating an atomic blast. The thick shafts of lightning didn't zigzag but plunged vertically. Occasionally, inside these wide shafts, bright flashes as thin as string zigzagged and plummeted into the water. Coleridge's *The Rime of the Ancient Mariner* flashed through my mind.

> The thick black cloud was cleft, and still
> The Moon was at its side:
> Like waters shot from some high crag,
> The lightning fell with never a jag,
> A river steep and wide.

Thunder, lightning, torrential rain. We were in the midst of a convulsion of the elements. Odysseus would have attributed this to the wrath of the gods. Was this our baptism of fire? Our initiation into what awaited us? Or our grand finale?

When Felix came up for his watch, I stayed with him till 1 am, then crawled into my bunk. But unlike Felix, who could sleep through anything, I couldn't sleep. The lightning and thunder, the downpour, continued relentlessly. We ploughed out of one storm and moved into the next. With dead reckoning and the GPS, we knew our position at all times, and we were fortunate the radar didn't pack up.

We changed watches at 4 am. When I came up, a ring of stars surrounded the moon in a pitch black sky. But when the moon moved behind a dark cloud, I was enveloped by an unimaginable blackness. I couldn't see the seat or the rail on the other side of the cockpit. I heard the sea rage, the froth pour onto the deck, the wind, the thunder. I felt water run down my face, my neck and my hands. I tasted salt. I was worried that claustrophobia would overwhelm me, but I didn't want to wake Felix again, so I moved close to the gangway and glued my eyes on the mini globe, a spec of red light on the radar. Instead of being terrified, as I always had been when caught in a storm, I was stunned into disbelief. This was so fantastical, so surreal that instead of being gripped with fear, I was fascinated.

Here I was, alone in the cockpit in a horrendous storm. It was black, still a long time till dawn. Why wasn't I quaking? Why wasn't I cold?

It was then that I felt myself float above the cockpit and look down onto my head. I felt I'd entered another world. The waves kept pounding. *Galatea* was tossing and I wasn't afraid.

Was this preparation for death? A message that I shouldn't fear death? Or was it a way to make a non-believer believe?

Then the clouds parted. A shaft of moonlight shone down the hatch and lit up Felix's sleeping face. It glowed like an eerie painting. And all around that face was blackness. As I gazed down, a strange, unearthly love for him welled inside me, and I licked salty tears.

I had no idea how long this lasted. Then I was back in the cockpit once more, my face streaming with tears and sea spray. How could I explain why, when sailing through previous storms far less violent than this, I was invariably terrified, and now I felt no fear? I kept my eyes glued on the tiny red globe on the radar as *Galatea* battled on gallantly.

Eventually, a pale pink haze appeared on the eastern horizon, followed by an orange disc rising from the sea. Then blackness faded to grey, and the day had begun. When Felix came on deck, I found it hard to speak. Exhausted and confused, I left him to it.

The rain, lightning and thunder had stopped, but the wild winds continued. As we neared Paphos, a notoriously difficult harbour to enter, I came up on deck. The visibility was bad.

'We may have to go on to Limassol. But that's 50 miles away, and we wouldn't get there in daylight.' Felix looked worried.

Then one of the many gods of the Eastern Mediterranean had pity on us. Twenty minutes before we were due to enter Paphos harbour, the visibility improved and we motored in.

'The mizzen's in shreds,' I said.

'She's given us a lot of use, we'll consign her as she deserves, ceremoniously to the sea.'

Tired and on edge, I was backing *Galatea* into the marina while Felix dropped the anchor, when a loud urgent WEEEEEEEE! wailed from the depths of *Galatea*.

Felix shouted, 'Keep backing for Chrissake!'

'I am!' I yelled.

When we switched off the engine, Felix diagnosed a broken regulator, which was overcharging the batteries. I patted our *Galatea*. 'Isn't she the most amazing wonder? Imagine if she'd broken down during the night?'

'I'd rather not.'

◎ ◎ ◎ ◎

Cyprus evokes vivid, deep-seated, memories for me. I was 7 years old, and on my way to Italy. We had set sail in the Lloyd Triestino ship *Galileo* from Haifa on the previous day, and arrived in Cyprus early the following morning. After the shock of finding out I was leaving my family and home for good, I'd been awake most of the night, in a state of panic.

At dawn I crawled out of my bunk and, although I wasn't hungry, I followed the smell of Arab food, which I loved. I sniffed my way to an outside deck where a group of Arabs, sitting cross-legged on the floor, were scooping food with pita bread from a plate. When they motioned me to join them I fled.

Later that morning, I saw them disembark and heard a woman tell the person next to her, 'They come here to buy wives. They pay for them by the kilo. The heavier they are, the better they like them, and the more they cost. They're cheaper here than in Palestine.' I still recall the relief I felt that they wouldn't want to buy me, because my grandmother had always said that I was much too thin.

I often wonder about conversations children overhear.

We spent some days in Paphos, then sailed on to Larnaca in search of a winter berth for *Galatea*. We were lucky.

'It's all fixed,' Felix said. 'They found a spot on the dry. She'll be well looked after. A lot of Brits live on their boats here during winter. They have all the facilities they need. They've organised clubs, even a bridge club.'

'That's great.'

'By the way, I've booked our flight to London. I'm looking forward to it.'

'Me too. And we'll be back here in April, then off to Israel.'

◎◎◎◎

For me, the idea of entering Haifa harbour under sail in our own boat was an emotional rite of passage, different from the many other occasions I'd flown in to visit my brother (with whom I hadn't lived since I was 7) and his family. Felix had no relatives there, but for me it was a return to my earliest roots.

It was a clear morning as we pulled out of Larnaca harbour the following summer and hoisted all the sails. With a steady 20- to 30-knot wind, froth curled and hissed at the bow, needles of spray pricked our faces and the wind whistled in the stays. The waves had built up and by lunchtime I was hanging over the rails. I swallowed more antinausea tablets.

'Go down, honey. I can manage on my own.' I crawled onto the bunk and lay flat on my back. From below I saw Felix's face. It was a shade of green. Soon after I heard him heave. He came down, took two tablets himself, and went back up. *Galatea* climbed up and rolled down waves.

By 8 it was dark and moonless, but the sky glittered with stars. The wind was steady; the only sound was our bow sweeping through the water, and an occasional shudder of sails. I climbed back into the cockpit, and we both stayed on deck all night.

In the morning, mist shrouded a pink dawn and hid the coastline. An Israeli patrol boat came alongside, accompanied us some of the way, and later waved us into port. The view of Haifa from the entrance to the harbour was unfamiliar. It didn't smell of hommus and falafel, my childhood recollection of seashore aromas.

Our arrival in port was not at all like the scenario I had so often imagined. We'd taken so many antinausea tablets we were close to collapse. Instead of brimming with enthusiasm when the family greeted us on the marina, we were zombies. The only consolation was that this was going to be a much longer stay than any previous one. We intended to spend time with family, and see friends we hadn't seen for many years.

One day I took a bus and walked on my own along the street where I'd lived with my parents and brother. My earliest memories were of a time when the street had been a new dirt road carved out of the side of the mountain. There were no gardens, and children congregated on the street — dusty in summer, muddy in winter — to play hopscotch, hiding, chasing, skipping, leapfrog, marbles…The atmosphere was one of warmth, togetherness and a shared sense of community.

Most houses were temporary wooden structures that took only a few days to construct. There was no electricity, and people used paraffin lamps and primus cookers. I can still recall the smell, and hear the 'paraffin man' calling out '*Neft!* Paraffin!', ringing his bell as he led a shaggy horse and cart down the street — always in the same loose shirt, dusty trousers and torn cap, always a grey sadness about his face. Later, when people started to build concrete houses and install electricity, he stopped coming. I wasn't as thrilled with electric light as everyone else. I loved the glow of a paraffin lamp, the flickering of the wick, the amber circle on the table, the shadow it threw onto the ceiling, the shapes that let my imagination run wild.

My parents and the parents of my friends had come to Palestine from Poland in the 1920s. They were all secular socialists, idealists with a mission to build a new country.

Materially, it was a frugal life, but for children it was rich and warm. If, on a rare occasion, a car drove down the street, we stopped to stare and see who was inside. Later, when the riots started, the vehicles usually belonged to the British police.

As I walked down the street some 60 years later, it was hard to impose those memories — of a time when everything was basic, new and clean — on the state of the street as it now was. It resembled a Third World country. Those clean, whitewashed houses of the 1930s were a dirty patchwork of splintering plaster, bare concrete, broken shutters and cracked balconies. The small yards were filled with household flotsam. My nostalgia was for long ago.

It was Friday afternoon the day I went there, and the street was bustling with people, carrying shopping bags and rushing home before the start of the Sabbath. Two disparate groups now lived there. The majority were 'black hats' or Chabad, the men with side curls, black suits and large hats. The married women wore wigs, as orthodox custom dictates, and had large families. The overcrowding in these small flats must have been daunting. Little girls wore long skirts, not shorts or slacks, and the boys wore side curls and yamulkes. The religious congregated close to their schools and places of worship. For them, this was a close, warm community.

The others who lived in this street were new immigrants from Russia, who were markedly different from the 'black hats'. Young Russian girls wore mini skirts, shorts and tops with bare midriffs. Most of the Russians in this street were poor, and many were old. The one-room apartment where my grandmother had once lived was now the home of a 90-year-old Russian woman. Her daughter, a professor in Russia, visited her every year. A soup kitchen had recently been set up in this street to help the aged poor. The need for a soup kitchen in Israel was something new. But then, the country has had to contend with massive immigration and defence expenditure.

Clothes strung on lines across small balconies waved in the breeze. A large dog, his paws on the ledge of the balcony, watched the passing parade on the street below. 'A large dog on such a tiny balcony,' I commented to a woman standing next to me. 'He's from Russia,' she replied. 'They bring their dogs and cats with them.'

Russian immigrants who now lived here moved into better accommodation as soon as they could afford it. A large number of them were engineers, musicians, mathematicians, scientists, doctors, dentists, nurses and a variety of other skilled and professional people.

I stood in front of the below-street-level apartment where I had once lived, where my mother died, and remembered it as it had once been. Small, new and clean. Now I saw a broken lamp, discarded pieces of furniture, and overflowing rubbish. It was too depressing, so I moved on.

While we were in Israel we visited friends who had left Australia in the late 1940s. They were idealists who had come to Israel to live in kibbutzim, and dedicate their lives to the communal ideal. One friend — once tall, good-looking and strong — was now hunched and in a wheelchair. His chiselled features were gloomy as he spoke.

'It's over 50 years since I left Sydney to come here and, unfortunately, things didn't turn out as we'd imagined. Many of our children have left, and most kibbutzim are in a bad financial state. We came here in our 20s, Dora and I are now in our 70s. I guess you could say we're disillusioned. Once we were the country's elite. But times have changed all over the world, and Israel now competes in the global economy. "High-tech" is now the country's forte, a different world from the agricultural settlements we belonged to.'

By the 1990s the fault line in the society appeared to be between the ultra-religious and the secular. Yet, in spite of the enormous problems of security, life went on. Tel Aviv was a buzzing place, where cafés, theatres, opera and cinemas were all alive and well, and the young were drawn there.

The most striking difference between Israel and the West was the youth. Compulsory conscription affected everyone aged between 18 and 21. In the army, the rich and the poor mingled, and were exposed to danger together. Here newcomers learnt to speak Hebrew. It wasn't unusual to see immigrant soldiers reading Russian newspapers. The army was a watershed in every young person's life. For their parents, this was the most worrying time of their lives.

We hired a car and toured the north. We especially looked forward to Jerusalem. We'd always loved its colours — the hills, the stone houses, the sunsets across the valley. There we visited old friends.

'We've lived in Jerusalem all our lives. I was born here. But the number of ultra-orthodox is increasing and the religious regulations impinge on our lives. Many like us are thinking of leaving Jerusalem. Sam and I haven't reached that point yet, but our children don't want to stay. They say that so many of the things they enjoy, they get in Tel Aviv, not here. Jerusalem is a wonderful place, but…well, what can one do? It's a pity.'

'The two months passed quickly,' Felix said when we started to organise our departure. 'We thought it'd be too long.'

'But I've now had my wish to sail into Haifa harbour. It's been a great summer and an emotional one.'

'It certainly has.'

We sailed back to Turkey and three months later put *Galatea* on the hard in Marmaris for the winter.

◎◎◎◎

The following summer we continued cruising in Turkey and anchored in the now familiar places. Each year there were more discos, more noise, but somehow, we always managed to find quiet bays, and continued to be enthralled by the beauty that surrounded us.

'Look at the seagulls gliding, do you think they're enjoying the silence?' I wondered aloud. We were sitting on the aft deck one late afternoon in Cineviz Liman on the Lycian coast, gazing into the luminous glow of an orange sunset. The water was the colour of burning copper, and the sky was streaked, as it often is after a three-day blow.

'I hope so,' Felix replied, looking up at the sky. 'It's hard to believe that this is the end of our ninth summer. We'll be back in London next week. We never dreamt we'd have so much time.'

'We've been so lucky. In spite of our problems, these years have been a gift so few people have. I wonder how many more...' I stopped there and tightened my arm around Felix. 'Look, there's the outline of a new moon over the hills. It's getting cool. Let's go down and turn on the lamps,' he said. The stillness was broken by the wake of two passing yachts, then we were alone in this deserted, silent anchorage.

◎◎◎◎

chapter thirteen

It was a brilliant autumn day and we were back in London.

'What do you think about going to Regent's Park this morning? I need to take photos for Tuesday's photography class,' Felix said, fiddling with his camera.

'What kind of photos?'

'Of people in different moods.'

'Great. I'll take a thermos of coffee and a book to read while you take your photos.'

Music drifted from barges gliding past as we walked along the canal path to the park.

Felix was quieter than usual. Now and again he stopped to snap people on barges, with drinks in hand. Londoners stripped to the waist and lay on the grass, in rented deckchairs, their eyes closed and their faces turned to the sun. Parents pushed prams, and children clutching boats collided as they ran along the shore of the pond. Young couples strolled arm in arm. A young man sat on the grass strumming a guitar. Tall poplars and London plane and yew trees had already started to carpet lawns with autumn colours. The park was crowded with people making the most of a warm Sunday at the end of summer. I had brought a blanket to sit on, a thermos of coffee, some chocolate and Zola's *The Debacle*.

A small boy with curly ginger hair and freckled nose clutched a black puppy and watched intently as Felix inserted new film into the camera. 'Excuse me, but would you like to take a photo of me and my new puppy? His name is Harry.'

'What a good idea.' Felix looked earnest. 'I would love to take a photo of you and Harry. And what is *your* name?'

'My name is Simon and that's my father over there,' he said pointing to a man stretched out on the grass. 'My mother is at home because she's looking after my new sister. Her name is Helen, but she can't talk yet.'

I felt a lump in my throat.

'You stand over there and I'll take a photo of you and Harry, and that will always remind me of you.' Simon's face was intense as he clutched his black puppy tight. As soon as the camera clicked, Simon rushed off.

'Wasn't he cute?' Felix commented.

'Yes, reminded me of David and Julie when they were little.' The lump was still there.

'Would you like coffee?'

'No, not really.' That was unlike Felix.

'How about chocolate? I found your favourite nougat.'

'No thanks, I've got indigestion.'

He walked away in search of suitable subjects before I thought of offering him one of the antacids I always had with me. I continued to read. *The Debacle*, this brilliant, terrible book about the Franco-Prussian War, was not the right book for me that day. Perhaps the surroundings were too idyllic. Why was I so restless, almost maudlin? Was it the memory of the kids when they were little so long ago? Was it the passing of time? Felix's unusual response to the suggestion of coffee? Apprehension? Something wrong?

I found it difficult to concentrate. When I looked up I saw Felix focus on four old people on a bench. All four faced the sun, their eyes closed, wrapped in woollens on this warm day.

When he noticed me watching him, Felix smiled and came over to sit on the blanket. He put his hand on mine, but didn't say anything.

'Shall we go for a walk? There's a fresh breeze and it's getting quite cool.'

'Where would you like to go?' he asked.

'How about the Rose Garden, we haven't been there for a long time. Or would you rather walk round the pond?'

'The Rose Garden I think, it'd be shorter.'

I looked at him. He looked serious. Declined coffee, chose the shorter walk — that was unlike him. We packed up and I took Felix's hand.

Petals drifted in the breeze like snowflakes, then coasted onto the carpet of grass below. The garden was a blaze of colours — yellow, pink, salmon, red. The scent of roses permeated the air and I took deep breaths, glancing at Felix. But he was somewhere far away.

'Well, that's the last of the summer roses.'

'Yes, it's well and truly the start of autumn.' The way he said it sent a shudder through me. Was this a metaphor for us? Yes, but surely there was still a long way to winter. He was unusually pensive as we walked hand in hand, and I slowed down to match his pace. The buzzing of bees was constant, peaceful.

'Puss, shall we go to the tube now? Before it gets too crowded?'

No answer. 'Puss, did you hear me?'

'What did you say?'

I repeated my question.

'Yes, it's getting late.'

I had never known him to be like this. Vulnerable. Withdrawn. His thoughts were miles away. Something wrong, but he didn't want to tell me, worry me. Maybe he'd found a lump somewhere. But when he had a recurrence of lymphoma he didn't feel weak, as if he had no strength. We crossed the Marylebone Road. After an afternoon of the scents of autumn, the fumes of vehicles were choking.

'Not much further to the tube, honey.' Felix was walking so slowly, I wanted to sound encouraging.

'Do you mind if we get a taxi?'

I was stunned. I couldn't remember the last time we took a taxi. Something was terribly wrong.

'Of course not,' I said, and locked my arm through his.

The back and underarms of Felix's shirt were wet. I resisted helping him take off his shoes. He lay down on the settee in the lounge and picked up the *Sunday Observer*. Still silent.

'Honey, I don't understand what's going on. You're so quiet, you walk slowly, you're not yourself. Tell me what's wrong. I must know!'

'Nothing much, I've got indigestion. I don't feel like eating or having coffee.'

'But it's not just indigestion. You've had indigestion before and taken antacids, it's got to be something more than that.'

'I'm not sure what it is. I'm very tired. Haven't been sleeping very well.'

'So what are you going to do about it? We'll be leaving for Sydney in a few weeks. You wouldn't want to feel like this on the trip or when we get there.'

'Well, actually, I also have chest pains. Maybe it's something to do with the heart.'

'The heart? Since when have you had chest pains?' My throat felt dry.

'A couple of weeks or so.'

'Why haven't you told me?'

'I didn't want to worry you.'

'Oh, honey,' I bent down, and put my arms round him. 'So what are you going to do?'

'I'll make an appointment to see a cardiologist. I'll phone around tomorrow.'

Suddenly I couldn't speak. What should I do? We didn't know a cardiologist in London. What time was it in Sydney? I wanted to talk to the kids. Stupid idea. Why worry them? Funny how when I had a medical problem I switched off, leaving decisions to Felix. He was always in control, thought things through, and decided what to do. But when he had a medical problem all I could do was worry.

Dr Little was a tall man with a firm, reassuring handshake. In his early 50s, he had thick dark hair, intelligent eyes and a ready smile. The room was impersonal, used by numerous consultants and furnished with the bare essentials. There were no stacks of journals, books or family photographs.

'Please, take a seat. Let me pull up another chair. Where do you practise, Dr Huber?'

'I was a surgeon in Sydney, but I retired quite a few years ago.' Felix gave him a brief résumé of our last few years.

'That sounds like an idyllic retirement. So what brings you here today?'

As Felix gave him details of his most recent problems, I realised that he'd been suspicious for some time that all was not well with his heart. He'd kept it from me.

'All right, you go in there, take off your shirt and let's have a look.' He motioned Felix to a couch in one corner of the room and pulled across the blue curtain.

I looked out the window at a tall elm. Its leaves — in shades of dark green, gold and brown — were wet. As I looked, I remembered our old gum tree in Smith's Creek. We had watched it change over many years. Branches had broken off; its tilt had increased, it had aged.

'Well,' Dr Little said after he'd examined Felix. 'I think I'll need to do an angiogram. Can you come into hospital next week?'

'Sure, no problem.'

I gave Felix a hug while a nurse waited to give him his pre-medication before the test. 'If you come back in a couple of hours, Mrs Huber, he should be back.' I watched as she drew a curtain around his bed.

Outside the skies were clear. Here and there fleecy clouds drifted past. It was warm again. A Qantas jumbo, a touch of home, passed overhead. Today I was optimistic, convinced that Felix was indestructible. He'd overcome so many problems in recent years. This would be no different, I assured myself. Was that because it was a warm, sunny day?

I walked briskly and crossed Wellington Road towards the shops and cafés in St John's Wood. I bought a paper, then looked into Restaurant Rembrandt. Whenever we wanted to splash, we came here. It was tempting, and with two hours to kill, I went in and sat near the window.

'An "opera" slice and a cappuccino, please.' I read the paper cover to cover. I looked at my watch. Time to go. At the counter I noticed Felix's favourite cakes — chestnut with raspberries. 'I'll take two of these, please.' Tonight Felix and I would open a bottle of wine and phone the kids.

Felix was in the last cubicle on the right. He looked pale and his eyes were shut. The blanket was up to his chin. I bent over, kissed him and squeezed his left hand. He opened his eyes, and looked disoriented.

'Honey, you're back in the ward. The nurse said Dr Little will be down when he's finished his list. She said all went well.'

He looked at me, almost his old self, and gave me a broad smile.

'I feel fine. What I needed was a good sleep.'

'Guess what. I went into Rembrandt, had a cappuccino and an "opera". Got two of your favourites to take home.' Felix closed his eyes again. I sat and waited.

'Dr Little will see you in about ten minutes,' the nurse said.

I felt my heart race and apprehension take over. Dressed in a grey suit, white shirt and a conservative spotted tie, Dr Little made straight for Felix's bed.

'So, how are you Felix?'

'I feel fine, but more importantly, tell me if you think I'm fine.'

'Well, I'm sorry, but you have two blocked arteries that need stenting. That explains your symptoms. I wouldn't suggest a bypass at this stage. Stenting works well for many people. Certainly you need something done.' He stopped and waited for Felix's reaction.

'Well,' Felix started after a long pause, 'not much choice really, so I guess we'd better go ahead. When could you do it?'

'I could put you on the list tomorrow. You can come in tomorrow morning, stay overnight and leave the following day.'

I felt a sudden chill and buttoned up my jacket.

Felix chatted animatedly all the way home. I couldn't speak. My mind raced. Nobody in the family had a history of heart disease. Felix had never smoked. He always exercised and ran up stairs. But that was no guarantee, I knew that.

As we passed Abbey Road, a busload of Japanese tourists packed the footpath, cameras glued to their faces. Crowds always hung about there. Beatlemania. We pushed past the animated laugher.

'Abbey Road, a temple to all faiths. Beats churches,' Felix said.

I just hung on to Felix's arm to reassure myself that he was still there. A small tree at the side of the road was laden with sprays of blue flowers. I picked one. It had a light scent that reminded me of the first perfume Felix had bought for me.

We were at the hospital early the following morning. I left Felix with the nurse. 'He's first on the list, and should be able to go home in the late afternoon,' she said.

When I came to pick him up, Dr Little reassured me. 'All went well, Mrs Huber. I ballooned two arteries and put in stents. This should solve Felix's problem.'

That evening Felix was unusually enthusiastic. Could it be the result of a better functioning heart, or plain relief? I wondered. Perhaps a little of both.

'Would you like to open a bottle of wine?' I asked.

'What's for dinner?'

'Chicken soup, God's panacea for everything, poached salmon, salad and poached pears.'

'OK, I'll open a white.'

After dinner I saw Felix look intently at the 'Travel' section of the *Observer*. 'We've often said we should go up the Nile sometime. This'd be a good time.'

'But we're going to Sydney in four weeks.'

'That's in four weeks, we could go before that.'

'Isn't that a bit much for you? In any case I'd rather go to Sicily.'

'I'd rather go to Sicily too, but this is the wrong time of the year.'

◎◎◎◎

Dear Kids,

Dad is well, if a little more frail than usual. He'd suspected heart trouble for much longer than he admitted to me. Another worrying time is over. All his recent tests are OK. And yet, although I haven't mentioned it to Dad, I worry about going back to the boat next year. Although the cardiologist said the ballooning and stenting should prevent an attack, I can't imagine what I'd do if Dad had a heart attack on the boat. I can't help worrying.

Dad's booked a ten-day trip up the Nile before we're off to Sydney. I'm not as keen as he is, but then he's pretty manic at the moment. All I'm looking forward to is to get home and see you all.

Two weeks later:

We're back from Egypt. It was interesting, apart from the fact that Dad had a bad chest and high temperature, started on antibiotics, was in bed three days, and missed the Valley of the Kings. Shall tell you more when we see you. Meanwhile I'll rush this to the post office.

Lots of love, Mum

As we waited for the luggage at Sydney airport, Felix's face was grey, he looked exhausted.

'Let me take the case off the carousel,' I said.

'No! It'd wreck your neck.'

'Well, let me ask that young man to do it for us.'

'No!' He was emphatic.

The family was in the arrivals hall to meet us. Emma and Jackie looked tall, slim and more grown up.

'Hey, Pop! There are great plans afoot for your 70th birthday party. We'll need to dig out old photos.' That was Julie at her most enthusiastic.

Some days later, Felix didn't feel well. He said he felt nauseated, and spent the morning lying on the settee in the lounge. Suddenly he called me. His tone was strange.

'What's wrong? You look in pain,' I said when I saw him.

'I'm having a heart attack, I'll call an ambulance.'

'I'll call.'

'No, I'd better call.' He got up, phoned emergency and spoke lucidly about what was happening. 'They'll be here in fifteen minutes.' There was no panic, no hysteria. He went back to lie down.

'Thank God we're in Sydney!'

'I guess so,' he muttered.

The ambulance arrived. 'Take these tablets, Mr Huber, they'll relieve the pain.' The paramedics rushed him to St Vincent's Coronary Care Unit.

'If you've never had cardiac problems until recently, then my guess is that it's due to the radiotherapy you've had to the oesophagus,' the cardiologist said.

I spent the following day with Felix as he was wheeled from one test to the next.

'We've looked at all the tests, Felix, and I'm afraid you'll need to have a bypass. We've put you on the list for Wednesday.' The cardiac surgeon was a tall, dour, laconic man. I started to shake. Although I'd coped with medical problems when the two of us were on our own, in Sydney

I relied on David and let him be the intermediary between Felix and the surgeon.

Two days later, Felix was wheeled into the operating theatre. I waited in a nearby room with a young woman whose husband was having a heart transplant. We were both silent and nervous. After some hours I noticed Felix's surgeon pass along the corridor. I ran after him.

'Excuse me, can you tell me how the operation went?'

He stopped, looking awkward and painfully shy. 'He'll be all right,' he said, and moved on.

'You can come into the post-op intensive care now, Mrs Huber,' the nurse said. The ward was new, and the sun was streaming in. Felix, looking pale and cadaverous, was hooked up to monitors, drips and tubes. I must have looked shocked.

'He's quite all right, Mrs Huber. They all look like that after the operation, but there's nothing to worry about,' the nurse said. 'You can sit down, it'll take a while before he wakes up.' I was grateful for the kind words, they reminded me of the kindness of the nurses in Montpellier. She moved on, 'Mr Smith, try to cough for me, come on…take a big breath…'

There was constant movement as the staff rushed from bed to bed, metal bowls clanked, monitors beeped and patients groaned. Relatives tip-toed in and out, doctors in operating gowns came and went, and patients were wheeled in and out.

A railway station, I thought, a life and death railway station. The man whose wife had shared the waiting room with me was wheeled in. He had a new heart. I wondered what it would be like to have someone else's heart. Did that make you feel different? He looked so young. A nurse pulled up a chair for his wife, who sat down and cried quietly by his bedside.

The recovery was a bumpy ride. Felix's pulse was too high and his heart was racing uncontrollably. I was anxious and depressed, and sat next to him in intensive care much of the time. But three days later he had improved and was shifted into an ordinary ward. A week after the operation he was back home.

'Thank God.' I burst into tears. Felix smiled. Subdued, he looked frail and had lost weight, but he was glad to be home.

'It's great to have family around, to be together. Three days to your birthday.' I gave Felix a hug. 'What sort of cake would you like?'

'The usual, of course, orange and almond chocolate cake.'

'Chocolate cake? Now, after a bypass?'

'You bet!'

When I opened the door on his birthday, Julie stood there with her two poodles, Jackie and Emma with their labrador, all three with ribbons and waving tails. It was a quieter birthday than had originally been planned. Only family. The day after Felix's birthday we started going on short walks. We had had to postpone our flight back to London by two weeks. I wanted to wait longer but Felix was adamant that we return.

I'd been thinking hard about the way we had lived during the previous nine years, and one day I broached the subject. 'Puss, we've had a long lucky spell sailing. I don't think we should test our luck too far. I wouldn't be happy sailing any more. I'd be too worried.'

He took a long time to answer. 'That's fair enough. I guess we'll have to sell *Galatea*.'

◎◎◎◎

'Under no circumstances are you to lift your luggage at the airport,' the cardiologist had told him. 'It's only four weeks since your bypass.' By the time we reached London, Felix was frailer than I'd ever seen him. Stooped, his cheeks caved in and black rings round his eyes, he coughed incessantly.

During the previous weeks I'd been surrounded by family. Now, I was aware how alone I was. Felix was quiet and hardly spoke. If he stays like this, I thought, I won't be able to cope. But when he'd recovered from the jet lag, he was more like his old self. 'I'm going to phone the shipbrokers in Marmaris, and tell them that *Galatea* is for sale.' I was shocked by the way he said it. As if he were selling a car. Of course I'd known that it would come to this. But I didn't want to hear the conversation. I didn't want to hear him say, 'Hello, Frank, Felix here…Unfortunately, we won't be sailing any more, I've had a heart problem…'

We were selling a piece of ourselves. *Galatea* wasn't an inanimate object. For us, she was real, alive. Selling her was like selling an old faithful dog, one who had protected us, welcomed us each time we returned, and given us joy, a new lease on life. It spelled the end of an era, an acceptance of the inevitable, moving along the conveyor belt that travels inexorably in one direction. I ran down the stairs and rushed out to the canal, to the barges. When I returned, Felix was placid and composed, reading the paper.

'Hi, honey.' He looked relieved, as if he'd shed a load. So different from what I'd expected. I fell into his arms. 'We've been so lucky…' I said, but couldn't go on.

'When we started, we thought we'd have two or three years. In fact, we've had so much longer…and knowing us, we'll find a new way to live the next few years,' Felix finished the sentence for me.

'There are some really good deals for Berlin. Would you consider going there?' Felix was looking through the 'Travel' section in the *Guardian*. 'I'll never forget the night the Berlin Wall fell. What times these have been! And we've been right here. Gorbachev, Perestroika, Glasnost, the end of the Cold War. What do you say, shall I see what I can do about Berlin?'

'It'd be interesting, although I'd rather go to Sicily,' I said.

'I'd rather go to Sicily too, but it's not a good time of the year. Too hot.'

'Yes, OK, Berlin. But you'll have to do something about your cough first.'

'All right, I'll see the GP.'

It took Felix a day to book a flight to Berlin, a car and hotels.

The guide, an intelligent young woman with long fair hair and lively blue eyes, wearing jeans and a T-shirt with 'Berlin the Erotic City' across the front, enjoyed showing the small bus-load of tourists her city. 'Berlin is a relatively "new" city, dating from the eighteenth century when it was the capital of Prussia. In 1871 it became the capital of Germany. After 1945 it was divided into four parts. Since 1990 it has again become the capital of a unified Germany. We'll visit the museums…'

In the late afternoon we walked by ourselves along Unter den Linden towards the Brandenburger Tor. Felix stopped suddenly. 'That's the Adlon Hotel, Hitler's favourite, where the leadership liked to get together.' He looked pale and tired.

'Let's sit down and have something to drink,' I suggested.

'Yes, outside. It's such a balmy evening.'

We found an outdoor café with cane furniture and pot plants. It was crowded. A waiter with a Slavic accent took our order. We watched the passing parade, sipped Campari and soda, and nibbled nuts.

'The people look so content. Look at the clowns, the street theatre…it's great. Like the 1920s revisited…' I commented.

'You know, I can't believe I'm sitting here in Berlin, 60 years after *Kristallnacht*. I remember it so clearly. I was 11, and I can still see Mum answering the knock on the door the morning after *Kristallnacht*, and seeing two Nazi officers. They'd come to pick up Dad, and take him to a concentration camp. They said they'd wait while he packed a small bag.

'I was standing at the dining table with my electric trains. Then, while they waited for Dad to pack his bag, they said they wanted to play trains with me!'

I'd heard that story before, but now it seemed to plague him. He needed to talk about it. I took his hand.

'The whole of the following week, Mum and I ran from police station to police station trying to find him, but we couldn't. Then one day he came home. Shattered. He'd been with hundreds of others, forced to do knee bends all day. On that morning the Nazis asked the people whether any of them had good reasons why they should be let go. They'd arrested so many after *Kristallnacht*, they didn't have enough trains to transport them all to Buchenwald, so they were prepared to release some of them. Dad happened to have the ship's tickets to Australia in his pocket, so he was freed, on condition that he was out of Austria within 24 hours. He left with a small group on the following morning and crossed the mountains illegally to Switzerland…

'I'd had a normal, happy childhood in Vienna, but that was the day I grew up. And now here I am, a 70-year-old man, sitting in a café in Berlin watching clowns and street theatre.'

I got up. 'Let's go, Puss.'

Hi Kids,
Berlin wasn't emotionally easy for Dad, in spite of the Pergamon, Nefertiti and the wonderful galleries. Too many traumatic old memories. After Berlin we drove

on to Leipzig. Hard to describe our feelings as we entered Bach's St Thomas Church, just as an organ burst into a cantata and filled the church.

Leipzig is so full of musical ghosts. Mahler composed his *First Symphony* during his two years there, and Schubert also spent time here. Mendelssohn started the Leipzig Conservatory and was director of the Gewandhaus Orchestra. A new Mendelssohn monument has been erected in front of the Gewandhaus, to replace the one destroyed by the Nazis in 1938.

The *pièce de resistance* was the concert we attended — Daniel Barenboim and the Chicago Symphony doing Mahler's *Fifth Symphony*. The audience went wild.

On the way to Dresden, we made a detour to Weimar to see, among other things, Goethe's house, which was supremely modest by today's celebrity standards. We hadn't realised that Buchenwald was only 8 km away. The people of Weimar supposedly had no idea what was going on there, although the street cleaners at that time wore the striped pyjamas of the concentration camp.

The inner town of Baroque Dresden has been almost completely rebuilt. So much to see — the Semper Opera, the Albertina, which was full of exotica collected by the Saxon rulers, the old Masters' Gallery in the Zwinger…

But this trip was very different from the kind we've been used to, when we spent days or weeks in one place, talking to people and getting to know supermarkets, banks, post offices, toilets, ship chandlers and markets. Shall tell you more when we see you. We were kind of tired when we got back to Blomfield Road.

Lots of love from Us Two

◎ ◎ ◎ ◎

The phone rang early one morning. It was Frank, our yacht broker in Marmaris, to tell us that *Galatea* had been sold. I thought we'd adjusted to the idea that our sailing days had ended. Felix seemed to take it remarkably well but at the end of that phone call I burst into tears.

Some days later, Felix saw me slumped on the bed, clutching my head, and realised that this was no ordinary migraine. I remember being lifted into an ambulance, hearing people round my bed, and someone shining a torch into my eyes. I heard '…it's probably meningitis,' and Felix reply, 'I'll phone the children.'

One morning I opened my eyes and saw Felix next to my hospital bed. 'How long have I been here?'

'This is the third day. You're better now. A neurologist has seen you and said it's meningitis. The kids wanted to come, but you're better now. Over the worst.'

The day before I was discharged, the neurologist, a solemn man with rimless glasses, came to see me again.

'Mrs Huber, you can go home tomorrow, but you won't feel like your old self for quite a long time. You were very ill.' During the following weeks, Felix did all the cooking and housework. The flat smelt of chicken soup.

'Puss, your culinary repertoire is getting so good you'll want to take over. Your chicken soup can compete with my grandmother's cuisine.'

But all this was taking its toll on Felix. His face was ashen, lined and thin.

'Puss, are you all right? Your cough, it's terrible.'

'The past few weeks haven't been easy. It's been a big worry, but you're OK now.'

'I have to be OK for our 50th wedding anniversary family get-together in Umbria.'

'It's another six months to go. But the Borgo di Bastia has confirmed the booking.'

We played at being upbeat.

◎ ◎ ◎ ◎

Dear Kids,

I'm sure you've wondered how we feel about coming home to Sydney permanently. We've thought about it long and hard, and decided that for as long as it's feasible, we'd like to spend six months of the year in London, and six in Sydney. Dad has lost much of his confidence, and knowing that he can no longer work would make being permanently in Sydney hard for him. Of course I haven't told him that this is my reasoning. We love the idea of living in London half the year, it's no sacrifice. I'm sure you'll understand. Meanwhile, I hope the history and photography courses will give him sufficient challenge and satisfaction.

His cough plagues him. He's been on different antibiotics but they don't make much difference. The fact that he no longer needs to worry about me may improve his spirits, but it's not going to affect his cough.

I'm sorry this is a short note.

Lots of love, Mum

We found we enjoyed spending more time than we used to in our tiny flat. We liked being close, just as we had been on *Galatea*. When Felix went shopping I looked at my watch. 'How long will you be?'

'I'll be back as soon as I can.'

'Don't be long.'

My illness had made us conscious of how close the call had been, and although we rarely articulated it, we thought more frequently about death. Previously, when death had been a possibility, we were defiant, and beat it. We felt a sense of personal triumph and returned to our life on *Galatea*. Now there was no *Galatea*, and with each day, our time became more precious.

Six months after my stay in hospital, when I still hadn't fully recovered, Felix found a lump in my breast. He didn't tell me until he'd arranged for an old friend, Michael Baume, a breast surgeon and professor at University College, to see me. Breast cancer had been in Felix's area of expertise, so for a short time he reverted to his old confident self and I was glad to let him take over. He and Michael decided that I should have a mastectomy rather than a lumpectomy.

'But what about our wedding anniversary, with the family in Umbria? We're supposed to be there in less than three weeks.'

'Don't worry, you'll make it,' Michael assured me. It hadn't occurred to him that we'd be mad enough to drive, not fly, to Italy.

I had the operation on a Wednesday and was home three days later. Felix had a supply of syringes to aspirate the fluid I was secreting in my chest. I surprised myself by how unconcerned I was. Perhaps this was because Felix was back in control.

Two weeks later, we left at 6 am to make the 10 am shuttle to France. We drove through a lush spring landscape of poppies, weeping willows and poplars. It was late afternoon when we reached Troyes and found a hotel.

'I'd better set up "theatre" to aspirate you, honey,' Felix joked as he brought out two white towels from the bathroom, spread them on the bed and set out his syringe, needles, cotton wool and spirits.

'They'll have fun cleaning out the rubbish bin tomorrow morning. We'd better clear out early before they realise they've had a couple of old drug addicts in the place.' We had a little energy left for laughter. We fled the hotel early and moved on to Tournus, where Felix set up his 'theatre' once more. But he was coughing and running a high temperature. He started once more on antibiotics.

We continued on to Aix-en-Provence, where he again went through his usual routine. 'Do you think they'll set the French secret service onto us? *Vieux Australiens* leave a trail of syringes and needles in one hotel after another?' I said. Felix was too tired to laugh.

It took us five days to get to Borgo Di Bastia Creti, a fifteenth-century farming estate in the hills of Umbria, set among pines and olives and converted into luxurious rustic houses. This was to be the grand splash we had planned for our 50th wedding anniversary. But when we arrived Felix had a high temperature and I was frantic. Julie and her partner Denise, Anne and David, and my brother and his wife arrived on the following day. By the time they'd all unpacked, I could no longer cope. I rushed into our bedroom and hid under the eiderdown. Felix came in.

'Honey, you'll have to come out,' he said.

'I can't, I can't face anyone. I'm exhausted.'

Felix's temperature remained high but he struggled on. He suggested to the others that they go sightseeing. We were relieved to be on our own, stretched on deckchairs near the pool.

One day during that week, we all went together to Assisi, on another day to Perugia.

On our last evening, we gathered in the central dining room of Bastia Creti for a celebratory dinner. The long table was decorated with spring flowers and candles. The doors opened onto a terrace and garden. Veiled beams of light shone onto stone tubs of cascading flowers. The chef, a rotund Italian, had prepared a festive meal. Zucchini flowers battered and deep fried followed by ricotta and spinach gnocchi with truffle sauce, osso bucco and vegetables, finished off with zabaglione. Tuscan wines flowed. After coffee and Vin Santo, we dispersed onto the patio. A shrill chorus of crickets trilled and a full moon hung low in the sky. I looked up and made a wish.

'I wonder where we'll be this time next year?' I took Felix's hand.

'Who knows?'

We were apprehensive about the drive back to London. By the time we'd realised that it had been madness to drive, there was nothing else we could do. We started on the *autostrada* via Perugia, Florence, Bologna and Milan, and on to Lago d'Orta where we planned to stay three days. Shortly after we arrived there, Felix's heart started to fibrillate, and continued for most of the night. He spent the following day in bed. I suggested we try to get someone to drive the car back to London, while we flew.

'No, another couple of quiet days and I'll be all right.'

After two days at Orta San Giulio, we set off and crossed the Simplon Pass into the Berner Oberland. Two days later we arrived home, thankful to have made it in one piece.

chapter fourteen

During the following months, Felix's cough was relentless. Whether it was the cough that progressively weakened him, or some other condition, we didn't know. At the Marsden, Dr Hunt examined him, but didn't find anything significant. He suggested Felix have more tests in Sydney. Felix saw a chest physician at a London teaching hospital who said, 'You'd better get used to having an old man's cough and being permanently on antibiotics. Your chest X-ray is clear.'

'What about doing an MRI?' Felix asked.

'You know what a fuss they make in hospitals about the costs of these tests. You need to fill in so many forms...'

When we left, Felix said, 'Never mind, we'll be in Sydney soon and I'll get all these investigations done there.'

'Don't try to take the luggage down, ask the taxi driver to do it,' I begged Felix on the day we left London for Sydney.

'All right. Just this time.' The fact that he agreed told me how he felt.

Tears trickled down my cheeks as we started our descent into Sydney. Below, city lights blazed like a fun fair.

'We've made it home,' I whispered. 'We're home.'

The family was there to meet us. At home in our flat, Felix collapsed into the big brown chair and beamed. We felt enveloped in warmth and joy. And although I didn't want the evening to end, we were beat. During the night Felix started to fibrillate again. He'd been fibrillating more often, and for longer.

'I'll book to have X-rays, an MRI, another full blood count and an appointment with the cardiologist.'

'Yes, the sooner the better,' I said.

His haematologist, Dr Dean, ordered a lumbar puncture and a bone marrow test.

David and I entered the consulting room with Felix to get the results of the latest tests. Dr Dean, a middle-aged man with a round, kind face, was behind his desk. His serious expression frightened me. My heart started racing. He picked up several sheets of results from Felix's folder. 'I'm sorry, Felix. It's not good news.' He took a deep breath. 'You have acute myeloid leukaemia.'

No beating about the bush. Straight and to the point. He was that kind of person. Although the words themselves didn't mean much to me, I knew it was disastrous news.

I'd always maintained that in these situations I wanted to know the truth. The entire truth. But now I wished I'd had more time to prepare. Prepare? I'd known for months that Felix's health was deteriorating. Felix must have known. But we went on with the pretence that his health would improve. For a long time I'd assumed the blame, convinced myself that it was my meningitis, the slow recovery, then the breast cancer and his continuing worry about my health that had reduced him to this state. I fooled myself that when I was well again, Felix would also improve. But in my heart I knew this was wishful thinking. After all, my illness couldn't explain the cough. Now it was out. There was a long, long silence. I didn't dare look at Felix.

'What would you suggest?' he finally asked.

'With a younger person, I'd probably suggest a bone marrow transplant, but…in your case, unfortunately, there is really nothing.'

The silences grew longer.

'How long do you think I have?'

'Probably about six months.'

I remember going out into the waiting room where Julie and Anne were waiting. I didn't go up to Felix to hug him. I didn't want to cry. I was numb. Felix's face looked more lined and furrowed than ever. His shoulders were slumped. When our eyes met, he tilted his head and gave me a sad, gentle smile and took my hand.

From there we all went out for dinner. That evening has remained a blank for me. I couldn't speak. I knew that this time Felix wouldn't take me aside and say, 'We'll work through this, honey, we always do. You and me, we always do.'

The following day, Felix phoned the haematologist who had supervised his chemotherapy before we had left for the Mediterranean, when he had had his first recurrence. After he'd spoken to him, he came into the kitchen and said, 'Warwick said he had a patient with acute myeloid leukaemia a couple of years ago who hung on for eighteen months and even went on an overseas trip!'

'Puss, we'll make it to Sicily yet. We've booked to go in March, that's only five months away.'

'You never know. You never know,' Felix said.

From then on, however, it was a downhill spiral.

In the early period, after that terrible prognosis, Felix had the occasional day without a temperature and felt better, but on most days I noted in the diary:

F. v.v.v. tired, coughing +++, has been put on more antibiotics.

In our 55 years together, there had never been a time when we couldn't talk. We had spent an inordinate amount of time talking. But now, I found it hard to communicate with Felix. He was silent. He had turned inward, cut himself off. I didn't know how to handle it. Some days I couldn't stop crying.

One night, when we were in bed holding hands, I said, 'Puss, we always assumed we'd go together. Either drown together or crash together. Now I want to go with you, but you must help me.'

He took a long, long time to answer. 'The kids would be upset...' Then, after a long pause, added, '...and anyway, you must write the book we were going to write.'

Was this his way of forcing me to go on, blackmailing me with the book? Or did it really matter to him? Perhaps a little of both? I thought about it for several days, then I promised I'd do it.

One morning when Julie was at our place, Felix mentioned that he'd love to see Broken Bay again. 'Let's have lunch at Akuna Bay restaurant. Get a table near the water.' He wanted to see the place, smell the gums and hear the birds one last time. And Akuna Bay was the closest we could get by road to our favourite Smith's Creek.

We parked the car in the parking lot across the road from the restaurant. With Julie holding his arm on one side and me on the other, we started to walk towards the restaurant, but in the middle of the road Felix collapsed. Cars coming from both directions pulled up. Two people helped us lift and guide him back to the car. Silent and shattered, we drove straight home.

The following day, we accepted David and Anne's suggestion, and moved to their place, near the sea in Austinmer, south of Sydney. There, overlooking the beach and Norfolk pines on one side, and the escarpment on the other, the scent of gums, olives, lemons, orange trees and herbs permeated the garden. Native bushes attracted flocks of sulphur-crested cockatoos, rosellas and lorikeets.

Felix sat silently for hours on the verandah, breathing the perfumed air, listening to the birds, the surf and the nightly chorus of cicadas. Wisteria and jasmine trailed along the verandah and birds of paradise swept down one side of the garden in a riot of colour.

David took time off work. Anne helped to look after Felix and did all she could to make him comfortable. Julie drove down from Sydney every day. Jackie and Emma were there much of the time. My brother came from Israel for three days to say goodbye.

One day, when they were discussing advances in surgery since he'd retired, Felix said to David that he'd love to see him repair an aortic aneurysm. This entailed inserting a tube through the groin artery and, using X-ray monitors, deploying the tube into the abdominal aorta.

So, on the following morning, Anne and I drove Felix to the hospital where, with one nurse supporting him on each side, he sat and watched David through a glass partition while he performed this procedure. Emotion overwhelmed him and tears ran down his face. He was too weak to stay to the end.

During his last week, Felix hallucinated much of the time, but was awake most of the afternoon of Jackie's twentieth birthday and tried to join in the cheer he knew would be his last family birthday.

It was a brilliant, soft day, the day Felix died. The sort of day he would have chosen to slip out to sea with all sails drawing. The sky was china blue, the ocean turquoise and smooth as velvet. On the beach, waves rolled onto the sand, frothed and slipped back out to sea. A gentle breeze ruffled the gums and silver olive trees. Butterflies fluttered from blossom to blossom. The scent of roses and jasmine drifted in through open doors and windows, and apart from an occasional bird call, one could touch the silence.

As I bent over to kiss him goodbye I promised to write our story. Then, with his gaze focused beyond the window, towards the sky and the escarpment, he raised an arm as if responding to someone or something, and breathed his last.

And as I gazed one last time on his still, white face, I relived the night of that terrible storm, when a shaft of moonlight pierced the enveloping blackness, shone down the hatch and glowed on Felix's sleeping face like an eerie painting. Then once again, that strange, unearthly love for him welled inside me and I tasted salty tears.

epilogue

Later that morning, David and I sat alone in the herb garden. A giant bright green and red king parrot appeared on a low branch on a nearby lemon tree. He sat motionless, staring directly at us for a long time. His fixed gaze on our faces was eerie. He frightened me. Then suddenly, he spread his wings and flew straight at us. We ducked. He just missed us, veered and disappeared. David had never seen that bird before and has never seen him since.

In the afternoon, two men in black suits came to Austinmer to take Felix back to Sydney for the funeral. They were Russian immigrants who had never driven down Bulli Pass or seen the views over the South Coast before.

'Zis is paradise on earth, for why did he leave zis?' one of them said.

Julie asked them to follow her car, so that Felix would travel one last time along his favourite route to Sydney via Stanwell Park. At one point, Julie realised she was running out of petrol and stopped at a tiny garage. When she came out, she was taken aback by the sight of two short, black-clad, rotund men, cigarettes in hand, gazing over the panoramic view of the ocean and steep coastline.

'Hey, Pop!' she exclaimed, 'Look at that sky, the sea, that coastline! Look, there's a long, black limousine and two Mafiosi. Pop! You've made it to Sicily after all!'

acknowledgments

◎ ◎ ◎ ◎

Of course I was going to write this book. I'd promised Felix that I would. But I needed the encouragement of friends and family to persuade me to try to have it published.

Arnie Goldman was the first to convince me. He spent hours going through pages I'd written, making comments and suggestions. Ken and Elaine Moon nursed me along and kept me at it by reading each chapter as I wrote it. I'm not sure I would have finished without them. I am also indebted to Eve Heller, Betty Raghavan and Agnes Selby for their comments. My family supported me, read excerpts and made suggestions. My son David went through the manuscript several times, and checked facts. Susan Hampton did a radical first edit and cut the book to a manageable size.

Some time later, I met Josephine Brouard, when I patted her dog Indy and told her that I suffered from dog deprivation. Apart from letting me take Indy for walks, she introduced me to Hazel Flynn, commissioning editor for Pier 9. And that was my good fortune. Hazel and my editor Sarah Baker have been extraordinarily patient and a delight to work with. I am extremely grateful to them and to the team at Pier 9.

Unfortunately, there is no way I can thank all the people we met during our peregrinations, strangers who went out of their way to help us. My thanks to them all.

aft the back of the boat; the *stern*

autohelm automatic steering

bar a long sandy shoal or a ridge of sand; usually at the mouth of a river or at the entrance to a harbour

boom horizontal pole attached at right angles to the lower part of a *mast*

bow the front of the boat

broad reach sailing not directly downwind, but still away from wind

cockpit the area to the rear of a sailing boat, where helmsman and crew sit

companionway the shaft housing the ladder that leads down to the cabin

compass the instrument used to measure direction

coordinates where the longitude and latitude intersect to indicate a particular spot

crosstree one of the horizontal spreaders or pieces of timber or metal that cross the *mast*

dead reckoning to calculate position by the boat's speed and direction

fairway the main channel used by boats in restricted water

forward front of the boat; the *bow*

GPS global positioning system; satellite radio navigation that gives one's position

head the toilet on a boat

headsail(s) the sail or sails in front of the *mast*

heave to turn the boat into the wind so it stops moving and doesn't drift

jackstay line, rigged along the boat, to which a safety harness can be clipped

ketch a boat with two masts (the forward *mast* is the taller one)

knot a measurement for speed: 1 knot = 1 nautical mile per hour

leads markers used in channels and at bar entrances to indicate the navigable channel

lee the side sheltered from the wind

log a written record of the courses sailed and other information

main the main sail on the *mast*

mast the vertical pole on which the sails are hoisted

mizzen the smaller mast at the back of a *ketch*

nautical mile unit of measurement used for distance at sea: 1 nautical mile = 1.15 statute mile = 1852 m

port the left side of a boat when one is facing the *bow*

roadstead an anchorage some way out from the shore

running sailing with the wind when the wind is from behind

satnav satellite navigation, which gives one's position

sloop yacht with a single *mast*

starboard the right side of the boat when one is facing the *bow*

stays wires used to support masts

stern the back of the boat

washboards boards used to close the *companionway*

way-points the points plotted on a chart when planning a route by sea

windward the windward side is the side of the boat the wind hits first

working sailing into the wind

yaw the movement of a boat when it goes off-course